DATE DUE

12-01-97			
10.18.05			

Demco

I.T. INTERVAL TRAINING FOR LIFETIME FITNESS

by Dr. Edward L. Fox
Dr. Donald K. Mathews
Jeffrey N. Bairstow

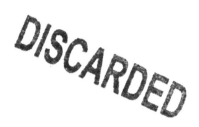

The Dial Press New York, N.Y.

A Bernard Geis Associates Book

Published by
The Dial Press
1 Dag Hammarskjold Plaza
New York, New York 10017

This work is based on a previously published book by Edward L. Fox
and Donald K. Mathews entitled *Interval Training*.

All photographs unless otherwise noted are by Tom Maloy and are
courtesy of The Ohio State University.

Illustrations #4, #5, #6, and #7 by Nancy Allison Close. #4 is from.
Sports Physiology by Edward L. Fox. Copyright © 1979 by W. B.
Saunders and Donald K. Mathews. Copyright © 1974 by Edward L. Fox
and Donald K. Mathews.

Manufactured in the United States of America

First printing

Library of Congress Cataloging in Publication Data

Bairstow, Jeffrey N
    I.T., interval training for lifetime fitness.

    Includes index.
    1. Exercise. 2. Physical fitness. 3. Physical
education and training. 4. Sports—Physiological
aspects. I. Fox, Edward L., joint author.
II. Mathews, Donald K., joint author. III. Title.
IV. Title: Interval training for lifetime fitness.
GV481.B2357   613.7   80–13518
ISBN 0–8037–4087–5

For Karen and Sarah

CONTENTS

LIST OF TABLES

INTERVAL TRAINING FOR LIFETIME FITNESS

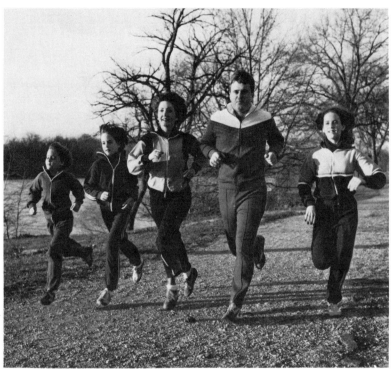

1. Every member of the family can get fit by using interval training—although the programs will differ for each person, one of the significant advantages of I.T.

1 YOU CAN BE FIT IN EIGHT WEEKS

Less Is More with Interval Training
It takes a lot of nerve to tell tough Ohio State football coach
Woody Hayes he's wrong, but one balmy fall day a few years
ago that's exactly what we did. Maybe he takes criticism more
kindly today, now that he's retired, but don't forget he was at
the height of his success then. What Woody was doing wrong
in his team's exercise sessions was exactly what you are probably doing wrong in your exercise program. Woody listened
to us because we are professors of physical education and
because he had heard about our remarkable breakthrough in
fitness programs. Here's what we taught Woody, and here's
what we plan to teach you too: With less exercise and more
rest, you will get fitter faster and stay that way with less effort
than with any other fitness program.

"How can that be?" you ask. In our research, we've proved
that the best way of exercising is to do it in short bursts with
plenty of rest in between. Running mile after mile for day after
day just isn't the best fitness program for most of us. We told
Woody to forget the six-minute mile as a training run for his
football players. Instead, we told him to use a series of 40-
yard sprints, with rest intervals between the sprints. Not only
did the team show impressive gains in fitness and was able to
sprint faster on the field during play, but the players liked the
program better because they no longer had to run that punish-
ing mile.

Our interval exercise programs will work with anyone, no matter what your age or present physical condition. At Ohio State we experimented with thirty sophomores who had never been in any kind of exercise program before. We divided them into three groups, giving each group a different exercise program. One group spent seven weeks in a recreational program that included swimming, scuba diving and golf. Another group took the tough physical education program that's used by the Army ROTC cadets at Ohio State, featuring such things as intensive daily calisthenics and grueling forced marches. The third group took an interval training —I.T.—program designed by us. That program had only three workouts a week, each one consisting of less than a half hour of actual exercise.

At the end of the seven weeks, all the students were carefully evaluated in our research laboratories. The results were astonishing by laymen's standards but no surprise to us. The

2. The principle of interval training is simple—work hard for a short period of time (*left*), then take it easy so the body can recover (*right*) before exercising again. (Photo credit: Stephen Szurlej)

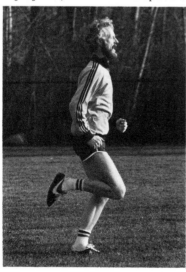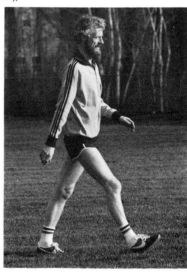

ROTC group was predictably fitter than the recreational group. However, the interval training group was way ahead of the other two in personal fitness—and this after only seven weeks and a total of less than four hours of actual exercise! Our tests also revealed another amazing fact: the seven-week interval training program had boosted the ability of the students to do hard physical work by more than 60 percent. We can do the same for you using interval training.

What Is Interval Training?
There's no big secret about interval training. It's simply a matter of exercise and rest. But here's the big surprise: Interval training means less exercise and more rest than other fitness programs. In a typical interval training workout, you will spend perhaps as much as two thirds of your time resting between quite short bursts of exercise. You'll work hard while you exercise, of course, but at the end of your training workout you'll feel much less tired than if you'd been exercising continuously.

Let's take an example. Suppose you were to run all-out for five minutes. You'd be near exhaustion, of course. The following day, run five one-minute intermittent runs at the same speed with one-minute rest intervals between runs. You'll be doing the same amount of work as with the five-minute continuous run. However, you'll be far less tired after the intermittent running. If you don't believe us, try it.

All our research has shown that the greatest enemy of physical fitness (outside of no exercise at all) is the build-up of waste products in the body as a result of fatigue during exercise. When these wastes build up, there's no point in trying to exercise further, but if you rest for a while the body begins to recover so you can exercise again. Depending on the exercise, recovery might take a few minutes, but even that recovery time improves as you get fitter from an interval training program.

You can use interval training with almost any type of exercise—running, bicycling, swimming, weight lifting, calisthenics, bench stepping and so on. You can even apply the ideas to any other activity in which you have to exert yourself. You can mow the lawn intervally or shovel the snow from your driveway. Maybe your neighbors will be puzzled to see you leaning on your snow shovel periodically while they labor away, but by working intervally you'll be finished just as soon. Furthermore—and here's the big plus—you'll be a lot less tired.

There's another key to successful interval training, and that's working a little harder every time you exercise. Each time you work out, you run, swim or bike a little faster or a little farther so you build up your capacity for exercise. In our programs, the build-up is deliberately gradual, so you'll barely notice that you're doing a little more each week. In eight weeks, interval training can take you to peak physical fitness. But you won't have to punish yourself to get there. You'll feel so good after exercising that you'll be looking forward to your next interval training workout with a sense of keen anticipation.

Nor will you have to exercise every day. We have proved that there's no benefit to be gained from exercising more than three times a week while you are getting yourself fit. There's no harm in the extra exercise, but you'll probably get bored by exercising daily. With interval training three times a week, you won't get bored so you'll stick to the program, just as our students have done. At the end of eight weeks, you should be fit enough so that even three workouts per week will be too much. We've found that you can stay fit with only one intensive workout per week once you have achieved your peak fitness. That's right—you need exercise only once a week to stay fit with interval training.

Can Interval Training Be Used If You Are in Poor Shape?

The answer to this question is a most emphatic "Yes." Interval training can be used by anyone. It has been used by older men recovering from severe heart attacks. Interval training is often used for training Olympic swimmers. Everyone can benefit from a properly designed interval training program. We'll show you later how to put together an interval training program that is designed just for you.

Recently, a Philadelphia businessman wrote to us, saying: "Last May I read an article about your interval training program. Having no interest in sports for recreation, I had, at age fifty-one, allowed myself to get into such poor physical shape that I could jog only about 100 yards without getting winded. . . . I began the program in June. After eight weeks, I could jog two miles quite easily. A friend who runs a mile a day on the RCAF program was surprised, when he ran with me, to find that his program did not give him the endurance that mine had given me. He is only thirty-six years old. . . ."

We were not surprised by this letter. We have had many others that praise the virtues of interval training. However, until now, interval training has been used mainly by athletic coaches. We know that the same ideas can be used by anyone who wants to get fit. That is why we decided to write this book.

When we say that interval training can take you to peak fitness, that's no idle boast. We have seen, time and time again, cases where interval training has completely changed someone's life. One of the most amazing examples is Jim Counsilman, the Indiana swimming coach. Jim has himself used the ideas of interval training for years with his college swim teams and as an Olympic coach. However, Jim devoted so much effort to his teams that his health suffered badly. In 1971, he was in such bad shape that his doctor told him to exercise or he'd be dead. At that point, Counsilman was suffering from asthma, arthritis, chronic bronchitis and high blood pressure. At 243 pounds, he was grossly overweight.

Counsilman began working out by using the same interval training methods he'd been advocating for his swim teams. He began gradually, of course, but eventually he could handle a daily two-hour workout in the pool. After nine months, he had lost over 60 pounds and had never felt healthier in his life. In the summer of 1979, at the age of fifty-eight, Jim Counsilman successfully swam across the chilly and choppy English Channel between Dover and Calais. He did it, Counsilman said, "to help lead a gray revolution to adult fitness."

We are not suggesting that you try for the English Channel, but we do know that interval training will get you fit so you'll be able to do much more without becoming fatigued. You'll relish physical activity because you'll do it intervally and enjoy it. The point is that interval training is not just for athletes. Even the person who has led the most sedentary of lives can start interval training now. You can begin interval training whether you are sixteen or sixty and continue with it for the rest of your life. Since interval training can be adapted to suit any person at any age, our methods are truly for lifetime fitness. Once you start an interval training program, you won't want to stop.

What Interval Training Will Do for You
When you get into your interval training program, you'll derive many benefits, some of which may not be so obvious:

- Your physical shape will be improved. Interval training will tone up your muscles so your sagging stomach will be flattened and your tired back will be straighter.
- Your heart and lungs will be stronger. Interval training improves the ability of the lungs to absorb oxygen and strengthens the heart muscles so they can pump blood more effectively.
- You will be able to control your weight. With the proper diet, an exercise program will help you lose weight while staying physically fit.
- Your stamina will be increased. Even though you may exercise for less than an hour a week, your stamina will improve so you can play an extra few sets of tennis or more holes of golf or work longer in the yard.
- You'll put more into your life. Regular exercise will make you feel better and less tired so you'll be able to attempt more demanding tasks in everyday living.
- You'll reduce the risk of serious illness. There's plenty of medical evidence to suggest that people who exercise are less likely to have heart attacks.
- You will recover faster from injury. We know that interval training has helped people recover more quickly from orthopedic surgery and bone fractures.
- You won't get bored by exercise. Interval training programs can be so flexible that you can substitute, say, swimming for running, or calisthenics for bicycling, so you'll never get bored by having to repeat the same exercises week after week.

But above all, you'll experience that soaring feeling of well-being that comes from simply being fit. There will be no struggle to get out of bed in the morning, no extraordinary effort to make it through to the end of the day. You'll be more alert as you go about your everyday business of living. And you'll wonder why you didn't get fitter sooner. You'll be feeling, and looking, so good that you'll almost be compelled to exercise so you never lose your new-found fitness.

Is Special Equipment Needed for Interval Training?

The most sophisticated piece of equipment you'll need for your interval training program is a watch with a second hand. During your rest intervals, we'll ask you to take your pulse from time to time so you can check on your own progress. If you don't know how to take your pulse, you'll learn later in this book.

Your heart rate is an indicator of how hard you are working during exercise and how fit you are. By taking your pulse just after exercising, you will be able to tell, for yourself, if you have been exercising hard enough. If you haven't, then we'll show you how to adjust your interval training program. This is one of the great virtues of interval training. You can adjust your program to suit yourself and you can progress in your program at a rate that you decide on.

Other than a good watch, chances are that you already have everything you need. If you decide that you'd like to run intervally, then of course you'll need proper running shoes and clothing. If you wish to bicycle, you'll need a bike and appropriate clothing. Our point is that interval training can be done without special equipment. You do not need a gymnasium to get the benefits of interval training.

Indeed, if you wish, you can set up an interval training program that can be done entirely in your own home or office. We have developed bench stepping programs that are used by Navy submariners in the cramped quarters of their vessels. You can use the same program in your home or office or even at the workbench. We could even devise a program for flight attendants using the stairway to the upstairs lounge in a Boeing 747 airliner.

Can Sports Be Used for Interval Training?

Almost any physical activity can be used intervally, provided that the effort is enough to make your heart and lungs work hard. Thus you can both train for a sport using interval training and use a sport for interval training. That may sound a little strange, but it's really quite simple.

We told Woody Hayes to use 40-yard dashes for his football players because the dash is more characteristic of the effort of football play than the mile run. If you are a weekend, high school, college or even professional athlete, you can use interval training to boost your sports performance. For example, tennis players need some fast footwork to get around the court and chase balls, so a tennis player's interval training program should have mainly short wind sprints. The wind sprints will help develop the muscles and the capacity to dash around the court. This applies just as much to the weekend tennis player as it does to the professional. In fact, the weekend player ought to use more interval training to prepare for his play since he will, most likely, play only on the weekends, whereas the professional plays much more frequently.

On the other hand, there are many recreational sports that can be practiced intervally. Racquetball is one popular sport you can practice on your own by hitting a ball against the wall and returning it for as long as possible. That will give you a good workout, but it would be better if you did it for a couple of minutes, rested for a few minutes, hit again for two minutes and so on. Practicing like this is using interval training that will not only get you fit but will also improve your racquetball play.

Even professional athletes are beginning to recognize the value of interval training. Sebastian Coe, the British track star who broke three world records (mile, 1500 and 800 meters) within a few weeks during 1979, credits much of his success to an interval training program designed by his father. The senior Coe, formerly a racing cyclist, understood the value of the sudden spurt when it comes to winning a race. So Sebastian Coe's running program consists not of the long-distance running done by other milers but of a series of interval runs around a track. Coe typically does six 800-meter runs at about 80 percent of his maximum capacity, with rest intervals of one and a half minutes between each run. This type of training has given Coe the ability to put out a sudden burst of energy at a critical point in a race. The result: three world records broken in a few weeks.

Will Interval Training Work for You?

We have seen interval training that has had a dramatic effect on the lives of all kinds of people, from the overweight businessman to the professional athlete. We know that interval training can work for you too, no matter what kind of exercise you have done (or never done) in the past. But don't think that interval training means fitness without work. There is no easy way to physical fitness, just as there is no easy way to lose weight. You will have to sweat a little, work hard and, sometimes, push yourself for that extra effort to get the most from interval training.

We do know, from our research, that interval training is the most effective way of getting fit quickly without wasting time or effort in unnecessary exercise. Our interval training programs can be designed to get you fitter faster than continuous exercise programs, but you will have to put the effort into exercising and staying with the program. However, we also know that you won't lose enthusiasm, because you'll feel better after each workout rather than totally exhausted. Nonetheless, the benefit you gain from interval training is entirely up to you. We can, and will, tell you what to do for peak personal fitness, but it is for you to work through your own exercise program to get fit. Remember it's your body, your health and your life we're talking about here. Interval training can help you make a commitment to fitness that will last you a lifetime.

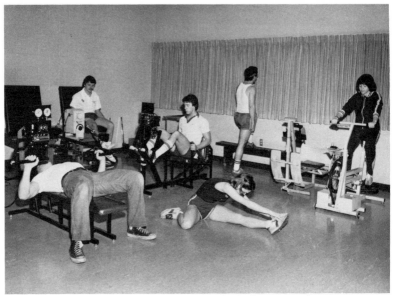

3. Virtually any form of exercise can be adapted to interval training so you can choose the exercises you prefer.

2 INTERVAL TRAINING AND HOW IT WORKS

The Best-kept Secret of Physical Fitness
John and Helen Dorsey, a married couple in their middle thirties, each jog a couple of miles a day at the recommendation of their doctor. Both started the program in roughly similar physical shape, although John, a former high school athlete, did have a slight edge. Helen, at her doctor's suggestion, jogged for one minute, then walked for one minute, then jogged for another minute, and so on until the distance was completed.

After a couple of months, their doctor tested the pair for endurance and general physical condition and found, to his great surprise, that Helen had moved well ahead of her husband in their friendly fitness derby.

That result comes as no surprise to us. More than ten years of research and testing have proved to us that by alternating properly prescribed periods of rest with exercise, people can actually gain more benefit from less total exercise. We know that a well-planned, personalized program of interval training can, after only eight weeks and a total of just over two hours of exercise (and six hours of resting between exercises), bring you to peak physical fitness.

Yet until recently, the idea of rest as a vital ingredient of fitness programs has been one of mankind's best-kept secrets. We'd like to lift that cover of secrecy for you and show you how to write your own I.T. program for lifetime fitness. First, we'll take a look at the way your muscles get their energy, because the chemistry of muscular energy is at the heart of the rest and relief principle of interval training.

How Your Muscles Get Their Energy

Whenever you move, many complicated chemical reactions take place in your body. Each of your muscles is like a tiny chemical power plant, taking in different fuels and using them to produce the energy that makes you move. Like an electric power plant that consumes coal or oil at a rate that depends on the demand for electricity, your muscles consume food and oxygen at different rates that depend on the demands you place on them.

For example, when you perform a sudden activity, like swinging a baseball bat, your muscles draw on a stored chemical called adenosine triphosphate (ATP for short). ATP is the fuel that your muscle power plant uses to generate energy. When you swing your baseball bat, your arm and shoulder muscles gobble up much of the ATP stored in those particular muscles. Fortunately, you'll pause for a few moments before taking another swing, which lets your muscles recharge with ATP and get ready for the next swing.

On the other hand, the store of ATP in your muscles is quite small, so this source of energy is good only for brief activities like golf and tennis swings or the 100-yard dash—activities that take less than thirty seconds (see Table 1).

Luckily, by the time your stores of ATP are exhausted, more ATP can be made from the breakdown of carbohydrates (sugar and glycogen), which are also stored in the muscles. The sugar is chemically converted into a substance called lactic acid (that same acid is produced in sour milk), releasing enough energy to make some more ATP. This second way of

The Energy Systems Used by Your Muscles

Work Effort	Performance Time	Energy System	Kinds of Activity
Anaerobic	less than 30 seconds	ATP	100 yard sprint, golf and tennis swings, base stealing
	30–90 seconds	lactic acid/ ATP	220–440-yard sprints, 100-yard swim, speed skating
Aerobic	1½–3 minutes	lactic acid/ oxygen	880-yard dash, gymnastics, boxing, wrestling
	longer than 3 minutes	oxygen	Jogging, marathon run, cross-country skiing, soccer

Table 1   When you work hard for a short time, your muscles get their energy without using oxygen (anaerobic activity). For longer-term activities, most of your muscular energy is produced with oxygen (aerobic).

making ATP—which we call the lactic acid system—will give you enough energy for longer activities, such as the 440-yard sprint (see table).

Naturally, there has to be a limit with the lactic acid system too. After a few minutes, the muscles that are working hard, and the blood, become saturated with lactic acid, and you'll

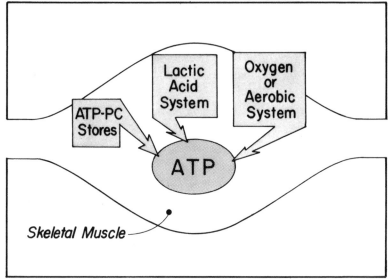

4. The currency of muscular energy is a chemical found in every living cell, called adenosine-tri-phosphate (ATP). Your muscles get ATP from three sources—from within the muscles themselves (the ATP-PC system), from the breakdown of sugar stored in the muscles (the lactic acid system), and from the conversion of food into energy (the oxygen system).

feel tired. The lactic acid produces a sort of chemical fatigue, although it is a very real fatigue: ask anyone who's just run a 440-yard dash! Of course, during rest or easy activity, like gentle walking, the lactic acid is eventually carried away from the muscles by your bloodstream and disposed of elsewhere in your body. The sugar in your muscles is replenished from the food that you eat. However, a properly designed I.T. program can increase the amount of both sugar and ATP stored in your muscles so you will be able to produce more muscular energy for short-term, high-intensity activities.

You may have noticed that we've said nothing about oxygen in all this, yet any physical activity quite obviously calls for faster and heavier breathing. That's because the energy produced by the release of ATP, either directly or by the production of lactic acid, doesn't require oxygen. The physiologists call those ways of generating energy "anaerobic," literally "without air." However, your muscles do need oxygen to start replacing the ATP you've used up. After a fast sprint, you'll end up with an oxygen "debt" that you must repay by breathing hard for some time after you've stopped running. However, if the anaerobic systems were the only ways of generating ATP, you'd never be able to run long distances. Fortunately, the same mechanism that lets you replace your ATP can be used to make more for longer-term efforts, such as jogging.

That brings us to our third way of making ATP—the oxygen or aerobic system. "Aerobic," as you might already have guessed, means "with oxygen." As just mentioned, your muscles store carbohydrates (sugar) and also fats. When either is chemically broken down aerobically, that is, in the presence of oxygen from your bloodstream, a lot of ATP can be made

5. The ATP-PC system takes phosphocreatine (PC) stored in your muscles and turns it into ATP for quick bursts of activity like sprinting or hitting a baseball.

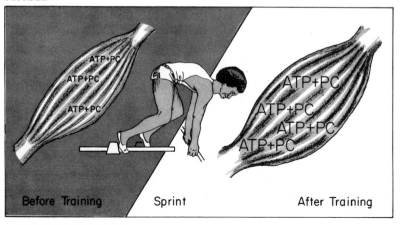

Before Training   Sprint   After Training

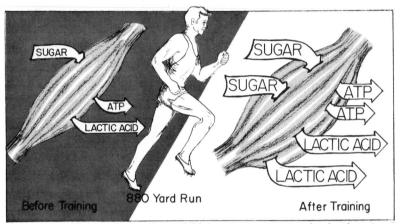

6. The lactic acid system produces ATP for intense activities that last less than three minutes, such as a half-mile run. Lactic acid is the byproduct of the conversion of sugar (stored in the muscles) into energy.

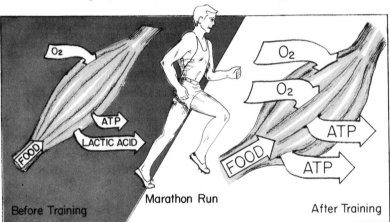

7. For continuous activities, such as a long-distance run, your muscles use oxygen (in the bloodstream) to convert food into ATP. The oxygen system is essential for man's continuous existence.

—far more than when oxygen is not available. However, the delivery of oxygen from the blood to your muscles is a relatively slow process. So the oxygen system starts slowly and builds up to produce ATP for such activities as long-distance running, swimming, skiing or even digging in the garden or shoveling snow (see table).

Just as you can design an I.T. program that will build up your muscular stores of ATP and sugar, you can also design a program that will benefit your oxygen system. We will later show you how to determine which systems, anaerobic or aerobic, you ought to work on and how to prepare I.T. programs that will improve one or both energy systems. But first, let's see how rest will actually help your muscles to do more.

Work and Relief—the Key to Interval Training
In the first chapter, we suggested that you compare a five-minute, all-out continuous run with a similar-distance run performed in one-minute spells with one-minute relief intervals between runs. We told you that you'd be less tired from the interval running. Now we can see why.

When you run hard for a short time, your muscles' store of ATP runs down (see Table 2). However, when you stop, the muscles start to recharge with ATP by means of the oxygen system, which breaks down carbohydrates and fats with the oxygen that you are breathing. The longer you stop, the more ATP you will replenish. In fact, with thirty seconds of rest, 50 percent of your muscular power is restored. Within two minutes, almost all your power is replenished (see table). If you run again for a short time, you will once more deplete your store of ATP. Of course, another rest will replenish your store, and so on.

The effect of all this is twofold. First of all, over a period of time the capacity of your muscles to store ATP will be increased, enabling you to do more high-intensity work. Secondly, less energy will have been supplied by your lactic acid system, so you won't accumulate as much lactic acid as

Your Muscles Recharge When You Rest

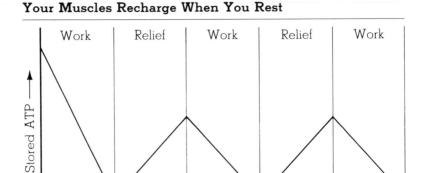

Table 2   When you rest during interval training, some of the ATP that was used as you exercised is replenished. That ATP can then be used during the next work interval.

Rest Soon Restores Your Muscles' Energy Stores

Resting Time After Exercise	Percent ATP Restored
Under 10 seconds	Very little
" 30 "	50
" 60 "	75
" 90 "	88
" 120 "	94
Over 120 "	100

Table 3   As little as half a minute is enough to put back 50 percent of the ATP that you'd use up in a brief but intense exercise.

in a continuous run. That means you'll be less tired from the interval running than from the continuous run. In itself, the savings you make in fatigue by working intervally will let you work harder. This is the key to interval training.

Just by exercising intervally, you'll be able to work at as much as two and a half times the level of continuous effort to reach the same degree of tiredness. Whatever your exercise program, you should do it intervally so you can do it harder for the greatest overall improvement in your energy capacity.

You may have noticed our use of the word "relief" instead of "rest" when talking about the intervals between exercising. There's a good reason for that. It's often preferable not to rest completely between bouts of exercise. In fact, we often suggest that the relief intervals consist of light or mild exercise. For example, if you wish to train by running, in your rest periods you might walk briskly or jog slowly. Although exercising during the relief intervals will slow the rate at which your muscles will replenish their ATP stores, there's a beneficial side effect. Your lactic acid system will get more use and so become more effective. Involvement of the sugar stores increases their capacity through using the proper length of relief interval and the proper amount of work during the exercise intervals. This is quite important for athletes who wish to train for events such as the 440-yard dash or speed skating, where the lactic acid system is used heavily.

So much for the changes in energy production that occur with the right I.T. program. Another important result is that interval training builds your heart's capacity to pump blood. Research has shown that the amount of blood pumped by each heartbeat is highest not during exercise but during the immediate recovery period from exercise. We also know that the more blood your heart can pump with each beat, the higher the capacity of your muscles' aerobic system. So when you exercise intervally, there will be many rest periods during which your heart pumps its greatest amount of blood. Thus, over the months of an interval training program, your heart's capacity will increase more than it would under a conventional exercise program.

There's one more fundamental idea in interval training that we haven't talked about yet. That's the principle of progressive overload. All that means is you must work harder as you become fitter. If you don't overload your muscles, you won't build up the systems that give them energy. Over the span of several weeks, your exercise program must grow progressively tougher to do you the most good. The I.T. program designed for you will have to change periodically so that you work harder as you improve.

The Basic Rules of I.T. Programs

There are six steps involved in constructing an interval training program that will be exactly right for you. They are:

1. Decide which muscle energy systems you'd like to improve—anaerobic (ATP and lactic acid) or aerobic (oxygen system). If you're an athlete, your choice will depend on the events you compete in. If you are more interested in general fitness, you'll probably want to improve all the energy systems, but with extra emphasis on the oxygen system.

2. Choose for your interval training program the exercise or exercises you most like to do. If you prefer running, swimming, bicycling, calisthenics or weight training, we've devoted special chapters to those activities to make the design of your own I.T. program easier. Those chapters have specific I.T. programs that you can adapt with little effort. If you'd prefer to use another sport, Chapter Eight will tell you how to go about it.

3. Select the rate and distance at which you must exercise during your work intervals. You'll need to make your heart work sufficiently hard as you exercise. That varies from

person to person, depending on age, sex, general fitness level and a few other factors. We'll show you how you can check out the proper rate and distance for yourself.

4. Decide how many work intervals you should have in each of your workouts. We've tried to group exercises into sets of work and relief intervals. For a runner, a set might be six 220-yard runs with rest intervals between each run. A complete workout might then consist of a set of 220-yard runs and a set of 110-yard runs.

5. Select the length of the rest intervals and decide on the kind of activity to perform in those intervals. The length of rest interval depends a lot on the intensity of the work that you do in your exercising. We'll show you how to select the relief interval and the activity that will go best with your workout.

6. Provide for an increase in intensity throughout the training program. As you become fitter, you'll have to work harder to keep on improving, although simply doing more and more quite obviously won't result in continuing improvement. It's not what you do so much as the way you do it.

In the rest of this chapter, we'll show you how to go through the six steps for yourself. In the chapters immediately following, we've gone through the steps for you and provided tables that you can adapt for your specific needs. However, you'll understand the tables better if you stay with us for the rest of this chapter, even if you eventually decide to use the tables in preference to working out your own I.T. program in detail.

Step 1. Which Energy Systems Should You Work On?
As we've said earlier, all three of your muscular energy sys-

tems can be used during some kinds of exercise, so we can't separate them out as neatly as we'd like. Let's go back to Table 1, based on performance times involved in sports and exercising. For each of our ranges of performance time, we've listed the energy systems used and given you examples of activities. We've also classified each group in terms of effort —anaerobic for activities that have performance times of less than ninety seconds, such as the 100-yard dash, and aerobic for activities with performance times longer than ninety seconds, such as jogging.

You can see that anaerobic effort involves mainly the ATP system for activities of less than thirty seconds or both the ATP and the lactic acid systems for activities of thirty to ninety seconds. Aerobic effort involves the lactic acid and oxygen systems jointly for activities of ninety seconds to three minutes and the oxygen system primarily for activities that last more than three minutes.

What does all this mean for you? If you are chiefly interested in general fitness, you should design an I.T. program that will put most of your exercise in the aerobic effort groups. If you are a sprinter, you should probably choose exercises that are mostly in the anaerobic effort groups. We'll be giving you examples of I.T. programs that can be developed for any of the effort groups or for combinations of the two areas.

Step 2. Choose Your Form of Exercise
This one's entirely up to you. As we've said, you can pick whatever exercise appeals to you or even switch from one to another as the mood takes you. If your major interest is simply in becoming fit, we've tried to make things easier by giving you more detail on running, swimming, calisthenics, weight training and bicycling in the following chapters. So your best

bet is to start with one of those five activities. However, if you'd prefer some other exercise, we'll show you how to go about designing a program in enough detail.

Step 3. How Hard Should You Exercise?

How will you know if you are exercising hard enough during your work intervals? There are a couple of easy ways to tell, no matter what the type of exercise.

The first is to check your heart rate by taking your pulse immediately after exercising. If you don't know how to take your own pulse, Chapter Ten shows you how. Table 4 indicates target heart rates for men and women at different ages. For example, a healthy twenty-year-old should exercise so that his or her heart rate is close to 190 beats per minute immediately after the exercise.

A second method of assessing your exercise regimen is a little less precise but no less effective. If you cannot complete all the work intervals in your workout, the rate of exercise is

Target Heart Rates During I.T. Work Intervals	
Age (years)	Heart Rate (beats/minute)
Under 20	190
20–29	180
30–39	170
40–49	160
50–59	150
60–69*	140

Table 4   Whether you are an athlete or have never exercised, you can check if you are working hard enough during exercise by taking your pulse immediately after stopping.

*Persons 70 and over should check with their physician before estimating a target heart rate.

too strenuous. On the other hand, if you can do more than the number of intervals you've chosen, the work rate is too easy. When you exercise, you'll soon learn the limits of your body and be able to adjust your work rate accordingly.

Step 4. Determine the Number of Work Intervals

Now let's look at an example of a specific I.T. program involving running and see how we can determine how fast and how much you should run. Each of our I.T. programs consists of sets of work and relief intervals. Let's take an example of a set that involves 440-yard runs (see Table 5). This set consists of four intervals where the work is a 440-yard run completed in ninety seconds, followed by a relief period of three minutes (twice the time of the work interval). If you were to follow this exact program as part of one of your workouts, you would run four 440s with three minutes of relief between each one. Each of the 440s would be run in ninety seconds.

A Typical I.T. Program for Running

	Work Interval		Relief
Number of Intervals	Distance (yards)	Time (minutes: seconds)	Interval (minutes: seconds)
4	440	1:30	3:00
one 440-yard run is to be done 4 times	run 440 yards	run 440 yards in one minute and 30 seconds	three minutes between each run

Table 5 This I.T. program suggests a set of four 440-yard runs, each to be done in one and a half minutes, with a relief interval between each run of three minutes (a total of eighteen minutes for the set).

This program was derived from guidelines that we have developed for running using interval training. We've summarized these guidelines in Table 6. You'll see that the left-hand side of this table is similar to Table 1. Now we've added exercise distances for runners and the work and relief intervals that go with those distances. Once you've chosen your level of effort, the table shows you the distances with which you should formulate your program, how many runs should be in each workout, the ratio of exercise to relief and the type of relief interval.

If you decide that you need a program with an anaerobic effort, you might choose to run the 220 in, say, 45 seconds sixteen times, with a relief interval that's three times as long as your running time (2 minutes and 15 seconds). The entire workout would take you a total of 48 minutes. Or you could mix up your runs by doing four 440s and eight 220s. In other words, half your workout would be 440s and half 220s, so you simply divide the runs allowed for each distance by two.

You can also make up a program from different types of effort. For example, you could do two 880-yard runs (from the aerobic effort group) and four 440-yard runs (from the anaerobic effort group). Your times for the runs would depend on your target heart rate, as was mentioned earlier.

If you are a swimming enthusiast, you can divide the running distances by four for the same type of workout. So you might write a program that involved, say, one set of two 220-yard swims and one set of four 110-yard swims, with appropriate relief intervals based on your performance times for the two distances. As the chart shows, the relief times would be three times as long as the duration of the swims.

We've also developed some guidelines for constructing I.T. programs on the basis of training times for such activities as calisthenics and weight training. We'll show you how to use those guidelines in Chapter Seven.

Guidelines for Writing Your Own Running I.T. Programs

Work Effort	Performance Time	Training Distance (yds.)
anaerobic	under 90 seconds	110 220 440
aerobic	over 90 seconds	440 880 1,760

Table 6   This table is the key to running I.T. programs. You pick your distances according to the type of program that you feel will best suit you. A jogger will select from the lower half of the table, but a sprinter will choose mainly from the upper half.

Step 5. Select the Length of the Relief Intervals

As we noted in the last section, our table of guidelines also tells you the ratio of work to relief intervals. Once you have found the performance times that you should achieve, it's a simple matter to calculate the relief times. For example, a runner who completes a 220-yard run in 40 seconds should use a 1:3 work/relief ratio, which would mean a relief interval of two minutes (120 seconds).

The work/relief ratios are based on the time required for your heart to recover and be ready for the next run or set of exercises. For example, for a twenty-five-year-old person the heart rate should drop to 140 beats per minute between runs (see Table 7). You can take your pulse periodically during the relief periods to check that your heart rate is indeed slowing to the right level.

What you do during the relief intervals is important. You can rest by walking about with some flexing of your arms and

Runs Per Workout	Work/Relief Ratio	Type of Relief
24	1:3	rest relief
16	1:3	rest relief
8	1:3	work relief
8	1:2	work relief
4	1:1	rest relief
3	2:1	rest relief

legs (rest relief), or you can engage in mild exercise, such as brisk walking or jogging. The latter we call work relief. Or you can do some combination of both types of relief. When you are most interested in modifying your lactic acid system,

Target Heart Rates During I.T. Relief Intervals

Age (years)	Heart Rate (beats/minute)
Under 20	150
20–29	140
30–39	130
40–49	120
50–59	115
60–69	105

Table 7 During your relief intervals, your heart rate should drop to the levels shown in this table before you start the next work interval.

you should use work relief. If you are working on your oxygen system, you should use rest relief to prevent lactic acid build-up during your workout.

Step 6. Make Your Exercising Stiffer As You Improve

Your workouts should become more intense as you progress through your program. You can do this by performing the activity more rapidly, taking shorter relief periods, doing more exercise, or some combination of all three. In the following chapters we'll show you examples of I.T. programs that progress on a week-by-week basis.

However, you can make the changes for yourself as you go along and you can progress at a rate that suits your own progress. One method is to measure your heart rate after you've completed your workout. Take your pulse a minute to a minute and a half after the last run or exercise of each workout. A lower heart rate after several identical workouts is a sign that you are improving and perhaps should be starting to work harder. Thus you can monitor your improvement week by week.

How Long to Get Fit?

When people begin an exercise program, they often want to know how long it will be before they are reasonably fit, or what is the minimum of exercise that must be done to stay fit.

If your main objective is general conditioning, an eight-week I.T. program with three half-hour workouts per week will bring you up to peak physical fitness. In other words even if you do not exercise now, you can become fit in eight weeks with a properly designed I.T. program (such as those in the following chapters). Increasing the number of workouts per week or increasing the length of the program will not bring about greater gains in fitness.

Once you have gone through an eight-week I.T. program, you should be able to maintain your level of general fitness by working out only once a week, following the same workout that you used in the last week of your eight-week I.T. program. With a once-a-week workout you can maintain your fitness level for several months. You should alternate an eight-week I.T. program of three workouts per week with a sixteen-week program of only one workout per week. This may seem like a very small amount of exercise, but we have tested the program and it works. I.T. can work for you too. All you have to do is stick to your program or to one of the programs that we recommend. I.T.'s up to you from here on.

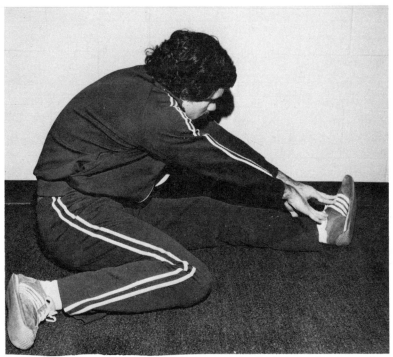

8. Stretching exercises are a must before any kind of physical activity—but you can do them intervally too.

3 WARM UP FOR I.T.

Take It Easy at First

No matter what the level of your general health or fitness before you start your I.T. program, you should go slowly at first. Although some muscular soreness is to be expected initially, by taking it easy you'll reduce the risk of extremely sore muscles and an aching body. Too many people drop out of fitness programs because in the first few weeks they go at them like a bull in a china shop. Nothing causes you to lose your motivation faster than a pulled muscle. So take it easy when you start out.

You can help your body to get used to the exercises by beginning every workout with a proper warm-up session. That way, not only will your muscles be warm and stretched, but you'll also be in the right frame of mind to put your best effort into the workout. Remember that much of a fitness program's success is in your motivation. If you like to exercise early in the morning, get up a few minutes sooner so you can move around, do the warm-up exercises that we suggest and generally wake yourself up so that you're ready to go. You'll find that you'll do the I.T. program much more effectively. And you won't be complaining about extremely sore or injured muscles, either.

Your warm-up session should consist of three kinds of activity: stretching exercises for flexibility; calisthenics for developing arm, shoulder and stomach muscles; and brief and easy activity of the kind that you'll be using during your workout. A warm-up session that has all three types of exercises will get your body ready to do its best in your I.T. program.

Get a Physical Before You Exercise

If you have previously been inactive or have a history of health problems, it's important that you check with your physician before starting an interval training program. Even if you are in good health, it's wise to tell your physician about your exercise program before you start, especially if you are over thirty-five years of age.

Your doctor should give you a thorough physical examination, which we think ought to include heart rate, blood pressure and electrocardiogram, at rest, during and following exercise. If your personal physician does not have the facilities to administer tests during exercise, he will be able to recommend a local hospital that should have the proper equipment. A full physical will cost $100 to $250, but it is money well spent.

We'll have more to say on this topic in Chapter Ten. For now, have your doctor check you out and get his or her approval for the exercise program you are about to start.

Stretch for a More Flexible Body

For most of us, our bodies begin to lose the incredible flexibility that we had as small children when we go to school regularly and sit at desks for much of the day. Later in life, we also spend too much time sitting at a desk or standing in one position in the work place. Our forefathers used to have much more active lives when they worked on the land. Even when traveling, they often used their own two feet. Now we sit in autos instead of stretching our legs.

A stiff and inflexible body can give rise to that familiar ailment of lower back pain, and a variety of other bodily aches. When you use muscles that have lost much of their elasticity, as for example in shoveling snow or digging in the yard, the danger of tearing a muscle or a tendon is great. So it's important that you do a variety of stretching exercises before you begin your I.T. workout. Don't omit them from your regular exercise program.

On the next few pages, we'll show you nine stretching exercises that should be done before your workout unless you are already doing suitable substitute exercises. You can select the exercises that you feel you need or you can do them all. Do each one about ten times, if you can, but do them gently for the first few weeks. And of course, you should do them intervally, with rest periods between each one.

The particular exercises we've chosen will help you increase the range of motion of a joint; will give you some insurance against stiffness and soreness and so reduce the possibility of a muscle tear; and will lessen the risk of tension in the muscles of your lower back, shoulders and neck.

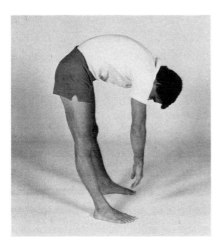

Standing Reaching. Stand upright with your feet astride. Bend at the waist with your knees straight and your arms and head hanging loosely. Reach downwards *gently*, relaxing your muscles and trying to touch the floor. (Don't worry if you can't at first!) Hold the final stretched position for several seconds. Good for the muscles of your upper back, buttocks, and legs.

Sitting Reaching. Sit on the floor with your feet spread apart. Reach with both hands first for one foot and then for the other. Try to touch your head and chest to the thigh of the foot that you're reaching for and hold the stretched position. Works on the same muscles as standing reaching, but does more for your upper back muscles.

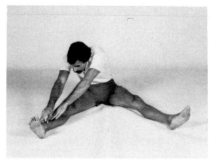

Trunk Stretch. Lie face down on the floor with your feet straight and your arms spread wide. Raise your chest from the floor, concentrating on arching the top part of your chest. Hold for six seconds. Good for people who have a tendency to slump, because this exercise stretches the chest and shoulder muscles.

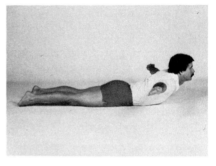

Alternate Toe Touch. Stand with your feet astride and your arms spread wide. Bend from your waist and touch your right hand to your left toe, holding the stretched position for several seconds. Stand up again and touch your left hand to your right toe and hold for several seconds. Good for the muscles of your shoulders, back, buttocks, and legs.

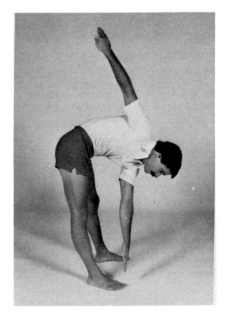

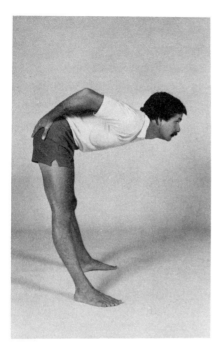

Waist Bend. Stand with your feet astride and your hands on your buttocks. Bend forward, keeping your head up, so that the top of your body is almost parallel to the floor. This is a fine exercise for the back and neck muscles.

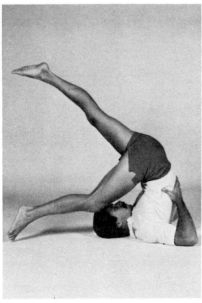

Overhead Toe Touch. Lie on your back and raise your legs straight in the air, supporting your hips with your hands. Point your toes and touch first one foot and then the other to the floor above your head. Hold for several seconds. Take it easy on this exercise at first. Excellent for the hip, upper back, and neck muscles.

Treading. Stand erect with your weight on your right foot. Place the ball of your left foot on the floor and transfer your weight to it gradually. Now transfer your weight back to the right foot. Gradually increase the tempo to a slow run. Good for flexibility and proper use of the ankle.

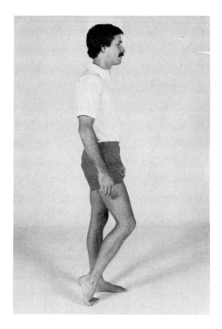

Chest Stretch. Stand erect with your feet a couple of inches apart. Hold your hands lightly clenched in front of your chest with your elbows bent and raised to the side. Keeping your head up, pull your elbows back and hold this position for six seconds. This is a good exercise for people with rounded upper back who need to stretch the back shoulder muscles.

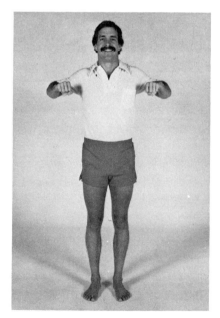

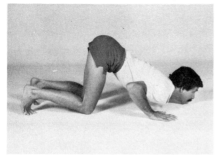

Spinal Stretch. Kneel on all fours and hunch your back. Bend your elbows, come slightly forward and lower your chest as close to the floor as you can. Return to your original position. This exercise will improve the flexibility of your spinal column.

Push-ups and Sit-ups for Strength

We think you should do two specific exercises in your warm-ups to strengthen your arm, shoulder and stomach muscles. Many people are weak in these parts of the body. You may be too. Push-ups will help you build up your arm and shoulder muscles and bent-knee sit-ups will strengthen your stomach muscles. Not only will these exercises build the muscles that you'll be using in your I.T. workouts, but they will also help your appearance and reduce the chances of low back pain.

You should do your sit-ups and push-ups intervally—we'll give you a guide that you can use with your eight-week I.T. program (see Table 8). If you find that our warm-up exercises are too easy, you can increase their difficulty by doing more of them (still within the I.T. guidelines, of course) or by making the exercise tougher. For example, you can do sit-ups on an incline or by holding a weight behind your head. We suggest that you do this only if you consider yourself an athlete and are already pretty fit.

You'll see that our guide provides for eight weeks—the time of our suggested I.T. program to get you fit—and has three sets of exercises for each of three workouts per week. On the first day of the first week, do two groups of eight push-ups in twenty seconds, with a one-minute rest interval after each group. That's a total time of two minutes and forty seconds for the push-ups. Next, do the sit-ups at the same timing, spending another two minutes and forty seconds. Time yourself with a

Push-ups. Lie face down on the floor, arms under your upper chest and your legs straight. Raise yourself up until your arms are straight. Hold for a count of "one" and then lower yourself gently to the floor for a count of "two." If you can't do a regular push-up from the floor, push up from a stool, the edge of a bed, or a staircase.

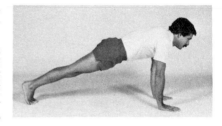

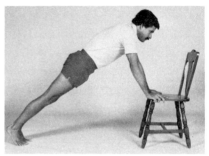

Sit-ups. Lie on your back on the floor, knees bent and hands clasped behind your head. Hook your feet under a low chair or have someone hold you by the feet and knees. Curl forward into a sitting position for a count of "one" and then lie back slowly for a count of "two." If possible, when you've become sufficiently flexible, touch your elbows to your knees in the sitting position.

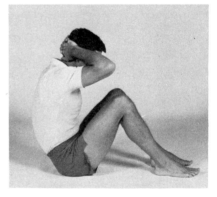

watch that has a second hand or do the exercises with a partner and time each other alternately.

You could, of course, do other exercises for your warm-ups. The I.T. prescriptions in our table could just as easily be used for any two-count exercise, such as pull-ups instead of push-ups, or leg raises instead of sit-ups. The main thing is to have a warm-up program and do it regularly before your full interval training workout.

I.T. Warm-up Program (for push-ups and sit-ups)

Week	Day	Sets	Exercises	Time for a Set (seconds)	Relief Interval (seconds)
1	1	2	8	20	60
	2	4	5	10	30
	3	2	9	20	60
2	1	4	5	10	30
	2	2	9	20	60
	3	4	5	10	30
3	1	2	10	20	60
	2	4	6	10	30
	3	2	12	20	60
4	1	4	7	10	30
	2	2	14	20	60
	3	4	7	10	30
5	1	3	16	20	60
	2	5	9	10	30
	3	3	16	20	60
6	1	5	10	10	30
	2	3	18	20	60
	3	5	10	10	30
7	1	3	18	20	60
	2	5	10	10	30
	3	3	20	20	60
8	1	5	12	10	30
	2	3	22	20	60
	3	5	14	10	30

Table 8

Do Some Easy Work to Begin

Before you start your I.T. program, whether it be running, swimming or some other exercise, you should do a few minutes of easy work using that exercise before you begin your workout proper. There are three reasons for this: preventing torn muscles; getting your heart and lungs moving; and getting yourself in the right psychological mind set to begin your workout.

Now let's take a look at our interval training programs for general conditioning.

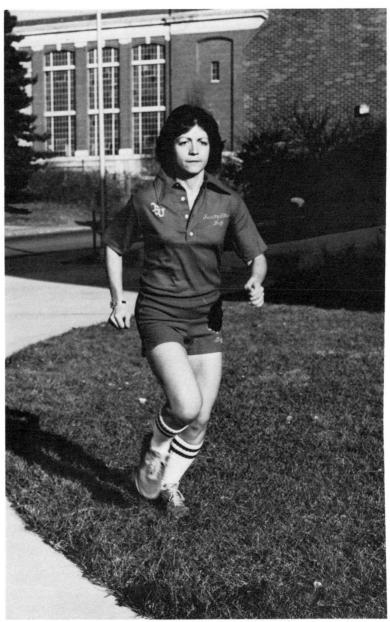

9. Running is the simplest exercise for interval training—from the casual jogger to the avid marathon runner.

4 RUNNING WITH I.T.

Running for General Fitness

Jogging and distance running have enjoyed an astounding boom in the U.S. during the last few years. It's a sport that can be performed by young and old, male and female, and it requires little more equipment than a good pair of running shoes. While it's undeniably true that running is a very healthy form of exercise, merely running a few miles every day or so isn't the best way to general fitness. Indeed, most runners are probably doing too much running, a factor that may give rise to ankle, knee, and back problems a decade or two hence.

The fact of the matter is that distance running—that is, of more than a mile—doesn't do very much for the anaerobic ways of generating muscular energy: the ATP and lactic acid systems. Not only that; running without intervals of rest is not exactly the easiest way of strengthening your heart and lungs. As we said in Chapter Two, your heart pumps the most blood during the immediate recovery period and there are many more of those in running intervally than in one long continuous run.

So whether you are interested in running to promote general conditioning or as training for a specific track event, running intervally will get you fitter faster and improve the capacities of your muscles' energy systems. Of course, it's important for the athlete to train at the distances he will run competitively, but that, too, can be built into an I.T. program.

In this chapter, we are going to show you how to use some tables of I.T. programs developed from the guidelines of Chapter Two. The programs are for general conditioning for both men and women for an eight-week period. We have suggested similar programs for persons in three different age groups—under thirty, between thirty and fifty, and over fifty years of age. These are programs for persons of average fitness. If you are of less than average fitness, you should progress more slowly than our tables recommend. If you are already participating in a fitness program or are of above average fitness, you can probably progress faster or make the workouts harder.

The Running I.T. Programs

You will see that our running programs allow you to make your own decisions about your running speed during the first two weeks. Instead of specifying a time, we want you to run at an "easy" pace. You must decide how easy that pace is to be. One running expert suggests that an easy pace is one at which you can carry on a conversation with a running partner. That's probably not a bad idea.

You'll also see that the program calls for three workouts per week for eight weeks (a total of twenty-four workouts over the length of the program). At the end of the eight weeks, you can change to two workouts per week for the next sixteen weeks without any significant loss of fitness. However, you may want to continue with the three weekly workouts. There's no harm in that, either.

No matter how you exercise, the first two or three weeks are the most important. The runs we suggest are fairly easy because you determine the pace that suits you best. This two-week running-in period lets your body adapt to the new stresses of regular exercise and reduces the risk of sore or torn muscles. During this time, you will also get to know your body in terms of what you can expect it to do (or not do) as you start running.

The first two weeks are the best time to start adapting our suggested I.T. programs to your own formulation. You are the one who is best qualified to write your own exercise plan. During your early workouts, check your heart rate, as we recommended in Chapter Two, and adjust the running distances or times to suit your own preference.

The programs we give in these tables are for general conditioning. They stress primarily the aerobic or oxygen energy system, but they include runs that will aid your anaerobic (ATP and lactic acid) systems. You can alter the emphasis if you wish by changing the distances (we'll explain how to do that at the end of this chapter in the section on "Training for Track and Field Events").

Remember, too, that these programs are for the average person in your age group. The overload progression of increases in the speed of running is aimed at the average person too. If you are having difficulty going from one week's program to the next, stay with the previous week for a few more days. Although it is an eight-week program, do not regard it as a rigid time progression. Of course, you'd be better off if you adjusted the workouts so you could stay with the progression at a lesser intensity. Similarly, if you find the going too easy, you should be working harder when you run. Adjust your running distances and times accordingly.

The best place to run is a measured running track. Check with your local high school or YMCA to see what might be available in your area. You may be able to find a football or soccer field that will be marked out sufficiently well to give you distance estimates. If you live in a city, you probably know that your city blocks are often a common distance. You can stride out a block to set up running distances for yourself. Alternatively, if your car has an odometer calibrated in tenths of a mile, drive a few blocks and measure them. In doing this, it's best to get help from a friend if your neighborhood is heavily trafficked. Let your friend drive while you measure off the distances.

How to Use the Tables

Our tables of I.T. prescriptions have been compressed to two pages for easy reference. As a result, the concentration of numbers may look fearsome but the use of the tables is made easier. We'll run through Table 9—the I.T. program for persons under thirty—so you can get the idea.

The table is arranged by week and by day within each week (the horizontal rows). Each block is one complete workout. For example, on the first day of the first week, we suggest that people under thirty run four 220s at an easy pace with a relief interval between each run that's three times longer than the time to run the 220. So if you run the 220 in forty seconds (a pretty good initial time, incidentally), your relief interval would be 120 seconds or two minutes. After the four 220-yard runs, we recommend that you run eight 110-yard runs, again at an easy pace, with a relief interval that's three times your time for the 110-yard run.

And so the week progresses. On day two, you should run two 440s and eight 110s. On the third day, run one 880 and six 220s, all at an easy pace. We again suggest using an easy pace during the second week. Of course, you should be checking your heart rate in the relief intervals during these two weeks and adjusting your pace to meet the target heart rates listed in Table 4, Chapter Two.

Running I.T. Program for Under 30s

Week	Day	Runs	Distance (yards)	Time for One Run (minutes: seconds)	Relief Interval (minutes: seconds)
1	1	4	220	easy*	1:3*
		8	110	easy	1:3
	2	2	440	easy	1:3
		8	110	easy	1:3
	3	1	880	easy	1:3
		6	220	easy	1:3
2	1	2	880	easy	1:3
		2	440	easy	1:3
	2	6	440	easy	1:3
	3	3	880	easy	1:3
3	1	2	880	3:00	3:00
		2	440	1:20	2:40
	2	12	220	0:38	1:54
	3	1	880	3:00	3:00
		2	440	1:20	2:40
4	1	2	880	2:55	2:55
		2	440	1:20	2:40
	2	16	220	0:38	1:54
	3	1	880	2:55	2:55
		2	440	1:20	2:40
5	1	2	880	2:55	2:55
		2	440	1:20	2:40
	2	16	220	0:37	1:51
	3	2	880	2:55	2:55
		2	440	1:20	2:40
6	1	2	880	2:50	2:50
		2	440	1:18	2:36
	2	16	220	0:36	1:48
	3	2	880	2:50	2:50
		2	440	1:18	2:36
7	1	2	880	2:45	2:45
		2	440	1:16	2:32
	2	16	220	0:35	1:45
	3	3	1,760	6:30	3:15
8	1	2	880	2:40	2:40
		2	440	1:16	2:32
	2	16	220	0:34	1:42
	3	3	1,760	6:30	3:15

Table 9

*For all runs at an "easy" pace, the relief interval should be three times as long as the time to complete a run.

Running I.T. Program for 30s–50s

Week	Day	Runs	Distance (yards)	Time for One Run (minutes: seconds)	Relief Interval (minutes: seconds)
1	1	4	220	easy*	1:3*
		8	110	easy	1:3
	2	2	440	easy	1:3
		8	110	easy	1:3
	3	1	880	easy	1:3
		6	220	easy	1:3
2	1	2	880	easy	1:3
		2	440	easy	1:3
	2	6	440	easy	1:3
	3	3	880	easy	1:3
3	1	2	880	4:00	4:00
		4	110	0:30	1:30
	2	6	220	0:55	2:45
		6	110	0:30	1:30
	3	1	880	4:00	4:00
		2	440	1:50	3:40
4	1	2	880	4:00	4:00
		4	110	0:30	1:30
	2	8	220	0:55	2:45
		8	110	0:30	1:30
	3	1	880	4:00	4:00
		2	440	1:50	3:40
5	1	2	880	3:55	3:55
		4	110	0:28	1:24
	2	8	220	0:50	2:30
		8	110	0:28	1:24
	3	1	880	3:55	3:55
		2	440	1:45	3:30
6	1	2	880	3:55	3:55
		4	110	0:28	1:24
	2	8	220	0:50	2:30
		8	110	0:28	1:24
	3	1	880	3:55	3:55
		2	440	1:45	3:30
7	1	2	880	3:50	3:50
		4	110	0:26	1:18
	2	8	220	0:45	2:15
		8	110	0:26	1:18
	3	2	880	3:50	3:50
		2	440	1:40	3:20
8	1	2	880	3:50	3:50
		4	110	0:26	1:18
	2	8	220	0:45	2:15
		8	110	0:26	1:18
	3	2	880	3:50	3:50
		2	440	1:40	3:20

Table 10
*For all runs at an "easy" pace, the relief interval should be three times as long as the time to complete a run.

Running I.T. Program for Over 50s

Week	Day	Runs	Distance (yards)	Time for One Run (minutes: seconds)	Relief Interval (minutes: seconds)
1	1	4	220	easy*	1:3*
		8	110	easy	1:3
	2	2	440	easy	1:3
		8	110	easy	1:3
	3	1	880	easy	1:3
		6	220	easy	1:3
2	1	2	880	easy	1:3
		2	440	easy	1:3
	2	6	440	easy	1:3
	3	3	880	easy	1:3
3	1	2	880	4:30	4:30
		4	110	0:38	1:54
	2	6	220	1:00	3:00
		6	110	0:38	1:54
	3	1	880	4:30	4:30
		2	440	2:25	4:50
4	1	2	880	4:30	4:30
		4	110	0:38	1:54
	2	8	220	1:00	3:00
		8	110	0:38	1:54
	3	1	880	4:30	4:30
		2	440	2:25	4:50
5	1	2	880	4:25	4:25
		4	110	0:36	1:48
	2	8	220	0:55	2:45
		8	110	0:36	1:48
	3	1	880	4:25	4:25
		2	440	2:20	4:40
6	1	2	880	4:25	4:25
		4	110	0:36	1:48
	2	8	220	0:55	2:45
		8	110	0:36	1:48
	3	1	880	4:25	4:25
		2	440	2:20	4:40
7	1	2	880	4:20	4:20
		4	110	0:34	1:42
	2	8	220	0:50	2:30
		8	110	0:34	1:42
	3	2	880	4:20	4:20
		2	440	2:15	4:30
8	1	2	880	4:20	4:20
		4	110	0:34	1:42
	2	8	220	0:50	2:30
		8	110	0:34	1:42
	3	2	880	4:20	4:20
		2	440	2:15	4:30

Table 11
*For all runs at an "easy" pace, the relief interval should be three times as long as the time to complete a run.

By the third week, we suggest the times that the average under-thirty person might achieve. On the first day, we recommend two 880s run in three minutes with a three-minute relief interval plus two 440s run in one minute and twenty seconds, with a relief interval of two minutes forty seconds. You'll note that the work/relief ratio is 1:2 for the shorter performance time. That's in accordance with the guidelines of Chapter Two. The remaining weeks are constructed on similar lines, with suggestions for the number of runs, the distances and times, plus the time of the relief interval. By the eighth week, your time for the 220 could be down to 34 seconds, and reduced similarly for longer distances. We must emphasize, however, that these times are merely suggestions. By now you have enough information to modify the running I.T. programs and to write your own plans.

During the relief interval for the running programs, you should walk around, flexing your muscles, or even jog slowly, keeping your body and muscles warm. If the day is cold, put on a warm-up suit so you do not cool down. As you get to know your body, you'll be able to tell how much you should do during the relief intervals.

If you are unaccustomed to exercise or if you exercise on a day when you are physically tired from other work, you may occasionally not recover from running as you should during the relief interval. If that happens, wait for your heart rate to fall to the proper level before you exercise again. If your heart rate does not recover properly within the relief intervals, stop exercising for the day. If you should overstress yourself, it may be several days before you can exercise again.

Similarly, guard against painful soreness, especially of the hip, thigh and the front of the leg. Continuing and painful soreness should be treated by a physician. You should not continue with your training program until the muscle has recovered completely.

Warm Up Before You Begin Your Workout

Even though you may have chosen to run as a way of getting fit, it's vital that you start your workout with a warm-up program. Follow our suggestions in Chapter Three and you'll derive much more benefit from your workouts. We cannot sufficiently emphasize the importance of a proper warm-up before any kind of exercise.

Use the Proper Equipment

If you have never run for exercise before, you should make sure you wear the appropriate clothing and shoes. There are many fine running shoes on the market today. We recommend that you go to a reputable sporting goods store and seek some expert advice on the best shoes (and socks) for you.

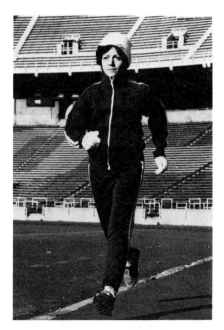

10. Proper clothing is essential for running intervally. In the colder months a warm-up suit, a hat, and gloves will keep your body warm during the relief intervals.

You should also wear clothing that's appropriate to the climate and season in your area. In the summer, shorts and a T-shirt might be all you'll need, but in the winter months a warm-up suit, a hat and even gloves might be necessary; you can always remove clothing layers as you warm up. We'll have more to say about heat and cold in Chapter Nine.

Run in the Right Place

You may have seen many runners pounding up and down the roads in your area at all hours of the day and even the night. We don't recommend road running for an interval training program. For one thing, roads are very hard on your feet and legs. Roads can also be quite dangerous when heavily traveled by cars and trucks. Further, it's very difficult to estimate the distances you'll be running in your I.T. program. Use the roads only if you have no alternative.

By far the best place to run, as we said before, is a proper running track at a high school or college. Not only will the surface be designed for running, but the distances will most likely be marked out for you. Check with the schools in your neighborhood. Such facilities are often available early in the day or after regular school hours. Some YMCAs now have jogging tracks too. As an alternative, you might consider using a soccer or football field. The length of a football field (including the end zones) is about right for many of the runs we suggest. Of course, grass isn't always in good enough shape for running, so you'll have to exercise some care when the ground is wet or frozen.

You might also check with runners in your neighborhood or with a local athletic club. People who are heavily involved in running will know the best sites in your area. Provided your running site isn't too far away, you can do your warm-up exercises at home, jog gently over to the track and be all ready to start when you get there.

For many people, running is an exercise that can be done in almost complete isolation and many runners enjoy that aspect of it. However, you may wish to do your I.T. program with a friend. The timing of each interval is easier if done by another person: you can time each other by alternating your running and relief periods. You may also get a psychological boost from having a companion. A little peer group pressure is a great thing for motivation, as many coaches know.

Of course, these same I.T. programs can be done by larger groups, such as a high school or YMCA fitness class. In that case, the timing might be handled by the coach and his assistants. The coach can also advise on the progression if he has a good understanding of the principles of interval training.

Training for Track and Field Events

If you wish to compete in track or field events, your training program should be based on the principles of I.T. For most events, a training program for the athlete will be different from the general conditioning program of the nonathlete. As an athlete, you should write your own I.T. programs, depending on the aerobic or anaerobic demands in your particular event. In Table 12, you'll find a set of guidelines for track and field events which shows the percentages of anaerobic and aerobic activity you should build into your workouts.

For example, if you are training for the 440-yard dash, your I.T. program should consist of approximately 80 percent anaerobic work intervals and 20 percent aerobic work intervals. This means that much of your I.T. program will be over the distance that you will race. Of course, you should also include some longer distances to build up your aerobic capacity.

As an athlete, you will be able to get better times for the

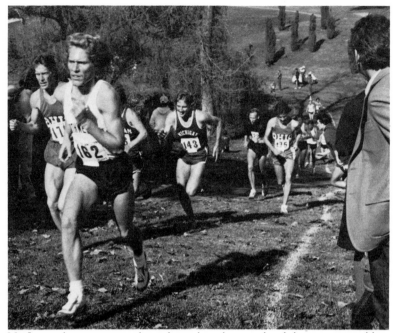

11. Interval training can be adapted to the needs of the running athlete whether for short or long distances.

running distances than are specified in our I.T. programs for general conditioning. So your times will have to be determined by you (and your coach, perhaps) to be sure you get a sufficiently intensive workout.

Track and field athletes might also want to incorporate weight training into their I.T. programs, especially during the off season for sprinters and field event athletes. The long-distance runner should of course continue to run during the off season, but cycling and bench stepping are also very valuable.

Proper warm-up is essential for all athletes to lessen the possibility of muscular injury. You can use the exercises of

Chapter Three, or if you wish to do something more demanding, try the warm-up exercises we suggest for athletes in
Chapter Eight.

Guidelines for Track and Field Athletes

Event	Percent Anaerobic	Percent Aerobic
Field events	90	10
100, 220 yards	98	2
440 yards	80	20
880 yards	30	70
1 and 2 miles	20	80
3 miles	10	90
6 miles (cross-country)	5	95
Marathon	0	100

Table 12   If you wish to train for specific track or field events, you should
choose your work intervals (see Table I) according to these proportions.

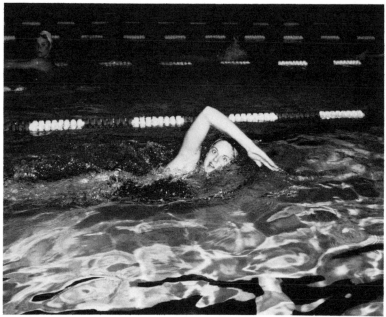

12. Swimming is an ideal exercise for interval training since most major muscle groups are used.

5 SWIMMING WITH I.T.

Swimming for General Fitness

Although running is generally the simplest way for the ordinary individual to get into shape, swimming can be just as effective. There is, of course, one big disadvantage to swimming—you need a pool. On the other hand, swimming is often more of a social activity than running. No doubt there will be others using the pool as you are training, and some of the swimmers may be exercising for general conditioning too. So you may more easily find an exercise partner than in the much more solitary activity of running.

Rather interestingly, swimmers, both long- and short-distance, have long recognized the benefits of interval training. Many school and college coaches use interval training principles for their swimming athletes both in and out of the pool. We'll take a look at the needs of swimming athletes later in this chapter.

Swimming does have one major advantage over running in that it exercises more of the major muscle groups. In particular, swimming uses the arm and shoulder muscles much more than any other popular sports except those that require special equipment, such as weight training, or certain conditions, such as cross-country skiing. Swimming also places less stress on the ankle and knee joints, which are often punished severely when one runs on unyieldingly hard roads. Swimming is often recommended for people who are recovering from muscular injury or who are susceptible to leg injuries.

If you are a high school or college student, finding a suitable pool should be no problem, though finding a time when the pool is sufficiently unused to allow you to train regularly may be difficult. For others, the YMCAs usually have pools that are excellent for training and indeed often set aside times or lanes specifically for people who wish to train rigorously. In many parts of the country, commercial health clubs and spas have fine pools and other facilities, although their membership fees may be somewhat of a deterrent. Your backyard pool may be too short for serious swimming. You could manage with a pool that's at least 35 to 40 feet long. Our swimming I.T. programs are based on a pool that's at least 25 yards long. You may need one that's longer when your training distances begin to improve. If you swim in a shorter pool, your times may be longer due to the extra turns you'll have to make.

You can, of course, combine swimming with other exercises to form your I.T. program. We know of a suburban Connecticut couple who cycle to the local YMCA, swim, have breakfast (provided by the YMCA for "early birds") and then commute by train to New York City. In the evening, they return by train, pick up the bikes and cycle home again. Not only have the pair improved their personal fitness, but they arrive in their offices ready to go for a demanding day of work. We've noticed that other city dwellers often drop into a pool or health club at lunchtime or on the way home. If you can do that, you should make a swimming I.T. program part of your exercise routine.

In short, we recommend swimming for your I.T. program as an alternative to running. Here's how you can develop your own swimming I.T. program:

Writing Your Own Swimming I.T. Program

You'll remember that when we talked about writing your running I.T. programs, we started with a table of guidelines based on running distances. That table can be adapted very easily for swimming, since you should swim roughly one quarter the distance of a run to achieve the same conditioning effect. It's just a matter of dividing the running times by four to obtain swimming guidelines. To save you a little effort, we've done that for you (see Table 13).

On our table of swimming guidelines you'll see that we've divided the swimming distances into anaerobic and aerobic exercises, as we did with running. However, it's very important for you to realize that these boundaries are quite flexible and depend largely on your own performance. Generally speaking, for those distances you can complete in less than ninety seconds, you'll be using your muscles mostly anaerobically—that is, without the supply of oxygen being a major factor. For those distances that take you more than ninety seconds, most of your effort will be aerobic.

When you first start swimming, you may well be unable to swim, say, 110 yards in ninety seconds or less, so a swim of that length will be an aerobic activity for you at that point. It's important that you use your target heart rates (see Table 4) as a guide when you begin your program. Adjust the times of your distances to get your heart rate up to the level we suggest. For example, if you are thirty-five years old, your heart rate should be up to 170 beats per minute immediately after your work intervals. At first, this heart rate may be reached after quite short training distances at very easy times.

For general conditioning, you should select 70 percent of your work intervals from the aerobic part of our table and 30 percent from the anaerobic section. For example, let's say you are at the beginning of a swimming program and you know

Guidelines for Writing Your Own Swimming I.T. Programs

Work Effort	Performance Time	Training Distance (yds.)
anaerobic	under 90 seconds	25 55 110
aerobic	over 90 seconds	110 220 440

Table 13   For general conditioning, approximately 70 percent of your swims should be chosen from the aerobic section of this table (lower half) and 30 percent from the anaerobic section.

that you can swim 25 yards in less than ninety seconds but you're not sure about 110 yards. Our table suggests you could do three sets of eight 25-yard swims or two sets of four 110-yard swims. Why not choose one set of eight 25-yard swims (33 percent of a complete workout), plus two sets of four 110-yard swims (50 percent of a workout)? You'll see that the percentages don't add up to 100 percent, but they're close enough for a start. Do these swims at an easy pace and use the rest relief intervals that we suggest—three times as long as your time for the 25-yard swims and twice as long as your time for the 110-yard swims.

You can balance out your percentages of aerobic and anaerobic activity over the three workouts that comprise one week's program. For example, let's suppose you've gone through several weeks of training and are now in your eighth week. Your workouts for the eighth week might consist of the following: first day—one set of two 220-yard swims plus two

Swims Per Workout	Work/Relief Ratio	Type of Relief
24	1:3	rest relief
16	1:3	rest relief
8	1:3	work relief
8	1:2	work relief
4	1:1	rest relief
3	2:1	rest relief

sets of four 110-yard swims (mostly aerobic activity); second day—four sets of four 55-yard swims (all anaerobic); third day —one 440-yard swim (aerobic). So you can see that the percentages of activity are approximately 70/30, as we recommended earlier.

If you'd rather not work out your own program, in the next section we will suggest specific swimming I.T. programs for various age groups. Of course, you can adapt these programs on the basis of your own performance too.

How to Use the Swimming I.T. Tables

The swimming I.T. programs in Tables 14–16 are constructed on the same lines as the running programs in the last chapter. As we mentioned earlier, swimming distances should be about one quarter the equivalent running distances for the same effort. So you could take one of the running tables and

Swimming I.T. Program for Under 30s

Week	Day	Swims	Distance (yards)	Time (minutes: seconds)	Relief Interval (minutes: seconds)
1	1	4	55	easy*	1:3*
		8	25	easy	1:3
	2	2	110	easy	1:3
		8	25	easy	1:3
	3	1	220	easy	1:3
		6	55	easy	1:3
2	1	2	220	easy	1:3
		2	110	easy	1:3
	2	6	110	easy	1:3
	3	1	440	easy	
—	1	4	110	1:20	2:40
3	2	12	55	0:38	1:54
	3	1	220	3:00	3:00
		2	110	1:20	2:40
4	1	6	110	1:20	2:40
	2	16	55	0:38	1:54
	3	2	220	2:55	2:55
		2	110	1:20	2:40
5	1	6	110	1:20	2:40
	2	16	55	0:37	1:51
	3	2	220	2:55	2:55
		2	110	1:20	2:40
6	1	6	110	1:18	2:36
	2	16	55	0:36	1:48
	3	2	220	2:50	2:50
		2	110	1:18	2:36
7	1	2	220	2:43	2:45
		2	110	1:16	1:32
	2	16	55	0:35	1:45
	3	1	440	6:00	3:00
		2	220	2:45	2:45
8	1	2	220	2:40	2:40
		2	110	1:16	2:32
	2	16	55	0:34	1:42
	3	1	440	5:30	2:15
		2	220	2:40	2:40

Table 14
*For all swims at an "easy" pace, the relief interval should be three times as long as the time to complete one swim.

Swimming I.T. Program for 30–50s

Week	Day	Swims	Distance (yards)	Time (minutes: seconds)	Relief Interval (minutes: seconds)
1	1	4	55	easy*	1:3*
		8	25	easy	1:3
	2	2	110	easy	1:3
		8	25	easy	1:3
	3	1	220	easy	1:3
		6	55	easy	1:3
2	1	2	220	easy	1:3
		2	110	easy	1:3
	2	6	110	easy	1:3
	3	3	220	easy	1:3
3	1	2	110	2:00	4:00
		4	25	0:30	1:30
	2	6	55	1:00	3:00
		6	25	0:30	1:30
	3	6	55	1:00	3:00
		8	25	0:30	1:30
4	1	4	55	1:00	3:00
		12	25	0:30	1:30
	2	1	110	2:00	4:00
		6	55	1:00	3:00
	3	8	55	1:00	3:00
		8	25	0:30	1:30
5	1	4	55	1:00	3:00
		12	25	0:30	1:30
	2	2	110	2:00	4:00
		6	55	1:00	3:00
	3	8	55	1:00	3:00
		8	25	0:30	1:30
6	1	4	55	1:00	3:00
		16	25	0:30	1:30
	2	2	110	2:00	4:00
		16	25	0:30	1:30
	3	2	220	5:00	5:00
		8	25	0:30	1:30
7	1	2	110	1:55	3:40
		12	25	0:30	1:30
	2	12	55	0:55	2:45
	3	2	220	4:45	4:45
		8	25	0:30	1:30
8	1	2	110	1:55	3:40
		12	25	0:30	1:30
	2	12	55	0:55	2:45
	3	2	220	4:45	4:45
		8	25	0:30	1:30

Table 15

*For all swims at an "easy" pace, the relief interval should be three times as long as the time to complete one swim.

Swimming I.T. Program for Over 50s

Week	Day	Swims	Distance (yards)	Time (minutes: seconds)	Relief Interval (minutes: seconds)
1	1	1	55	easy*	1:3*
		4	25	easy	1:3
	2	1	55	easy	1:3
		4	25	easy	1:3
	3	1	55	easy	1:3
		4	25	easy	1:3
2	1	2	55	easy	1:3
		4	25	easy	1:3
	2	2	55	easy	1:3
		4	25	easy	1:3
	3	2	55	easy	1:3
		4	25	easy	1:3
3	1	1	110	4:00	8:00
		4	25	1:00	3:00
	2	2	55	2:00	6:00
		4	25	1:00	3:00
	3	1	110	4:00	8:00
		4	25	1:00	3:00
4	1	2	110	3:40	7:20
		4	25	1:00	3:00
	2	2	55	1:50	5:30
		4	25	1:00	3:00
	3	2	110	3:40	7:20
		4	25	1:00	3:00
5	1	2	110	3:20	6:40
		6	25	0:50	2:30
	2	4	55	1:40	5:00
		4	25	0:50	2:30
	3	2	110	3:20	6:40
		6	25	0:50	2:30
6	1	2	110	3:00	6:00
		6	25	0:45	2:15
	2	4	55	1:30	4:30
		4	25	0:45	2:15
	3	2	110	3:00	6:00
		6	25	0:45	2:15
7	1	2	110	2:45	5:30
		8	25	0:40	2:00
	2	4	55	1:20	4:00
		8	25	0:40	2:00
	3	2	110	2:45	5:30
		8	25	0:40	2:00
8	1	2	110	2:30	5:00
		8	25	0:35	1:45
	2	4	55	1:15	3:45
		8	25	0:35	1:45
	3	2	110	2:30	5:00
		8	25	0:35	1:45

Table 16

*For all swims at an "easy" pace, the relief interval should be three times as long as the time to complete one swim.

divide all the distances by four to arrive at a similar set of charts. However, we have made some modifications of the tables based on our experience with college men and women swimmers.

We are assuming that you will swim free-style, since that is usually the fastest stroke for most people. However, if you prefer to use another stroke, you can do so. Simply use the same training distances, but remember that your times will be slower. You will have to adjust the times based on your own measurements of your heart rate. Naturally, you can swim part of your program with one stroke and part with another. Some people find swimming up and down the length of a pool to be somewhat boring. If using several strokes stops you from getting bored, by all means put them in your program.

You'll notice that we do not suggest any training times for the workouts during the first two weeks. We simply say that you must take the distances at an "easy" pace. What is easy? That's up to you. Quite obviously, an easy pace for a college athlete is far different from that of a fifty-year-old man who is starting an exercise program for the first time in his life. During those first two weeks, take your heart rate several times during your workout; most large pools have a big clock with a second hand that you can use for timing your pulse. Adjust your pace to meet the target heart rates listed in Table 4.

As with our running programs, the swimming I.T. programs are arranged by week and by day within each week (the horizontal rows). Each block is one complete workout. For example, on the first day of the first week of the program for the Under 30s, we suggest one set of four 55-yard swims, followed by one set of eight 25-yard swims. Each swim should be followed by a rest interval that's three times as long as the time taken for the swim. So if you take one minute for a 55-yard swim, you must then rest for three minutes.

Starting with the third week, our tables indicate the possible times you might aim for. Again, we stress that these times are merely our suggestions. If the pace is too slow, you can go faster to achieve your target heart rate. Similarly, if the workouts seem too strenuous, slow down your times until you get things under control.

During the relief intervals, you can paddle around or swim slowly. There's no advantage in getting out of the pool and taking your rest by walking around. For the middle distances (110 yards), we think some form of work relief should be done. In swimming, all this means is that you should swim slowly during the rest interval. Don't swim too hard or you'll not be ready for your next work interval.

Remember to check your heart rate from time to time as you progress from week to week. Some days, your heart may not recover as quickly as it should during your rest intervals. There are a variety of reasons for that, of course: you may be overtired or you may be doing too much exercise. Whatever the reason, wait for your heart to slow down before you exercise again. If your heart is not recovering properly during the rest intervals, stop exercising for the day. If you overstress your cardiovascular system, it may be several days before you can resume regular exercise. Of course, if you experience continuing difficulty with high heart rates, you must consult your physician before going any further. Your body will often give you early warning signals during an exercise program. Make sure that you heed those signals and get professional help from your physician.

Swimming and Running I.T. Programs

We mentioned earlier the suburban couple who bike and swim before commuting to work. Just as they mix cycling and swimming, you can devise an I.T. program of running and swimming. If you'd prefer to use your bike, we'll show you some cycling programs later on, in Chapter Six.

Since the running (see Table 6) and swimming guidelines are based on the same tables, you can mix the two activities by simple substitution. You'll remember that we said swimming distances are approximately one fourth the running distances for the same work effort. Thus a 55-yard swim is equivalent to a 220-yard run. So if your I.T. program calls for, say, a workout of two 220-yard swims and two 110-yard swims, you could do two 880-yard runs and two 110-yard swims.

One of us (JNB) lives on the Connecticut shore a little more than half a mile from the beach. So an excellent summer workout is to run to the beach, swim and then run back home —with appropriate rest intervals, of course. Such a workout seems much more of a pleasure than a chore, particularly after a hard day's work. And that is one of the great advantages of the interval training method: you can make adjustments in your program to suit your own needs and the dictates of circumstance.

On your vacation, you can mix running and swimming quite easily too. For example, if your workout normally calls for, say, four sets of four 220-yard runs on one day, you could run four 220s along the beach, swim four 55s (one quarter of your normal 220) and so on. Be cautious about swimming in the sea, however, since currents can affect your training times quite seriously.

This flexibility of I.T. programs is very useful if your days do not fit into a regular routine or if your work calls for much travel away from home base. Should you be in a place where you cannot run, such as a heavily polluted city on a day of high heat and humidity, seek out a pool and swim instead of run. Naturally, your swimming times will not be as good as your regular running times for the equivalent distances. Don't worry about that: it's far better that you stick with an I.T. program than miss a few workouts because of travel or other commitments. Once you become truly involved in exercise as a way of life, you will find ways to maintain your fitness program. It is one of the great advantages of I.T. that you can continually modify your own training program to fit your own circumstances.

Training for Swimming Events

For swimming athletes, a training program based on the principles of I.T. will, naturally, depend on the particular event or events you wish to enter. However, it is a simple matter to write out your own I.T. programs. We've analyzed the degree to which each swimming event makes use of anaerobic and aerobic muscular effort. In Table 17, we present a listing of percentages from which you can write your own I.T. programs using the guidelines we gave you earlier for general conditioning using swimming (see Table 13).

For example, if you are in training for 100-yard events, your

Guidelines for Swimming Athletes

Event	Percent Anaerobic	Percent Aerobic
diving	98	2
50 yards	98	2
100 yards	80	20
200 yards	40	60
400, 500 yards	20	80
1500 yards, 1500 meters	10	90

Table 17 If you wish to train for a specific swimming event, you should choose your work intervals (see Table I) according to these proportions.

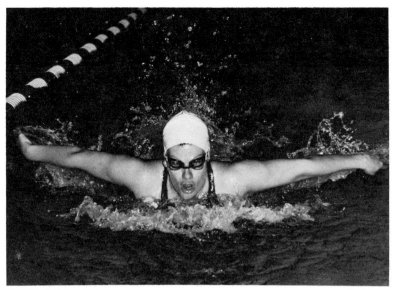

13. The ideas of interval training have been used successfully to train Olympic-class swimmers.

I.T. program should consist of approximately 80 percent anaerobic work intervals and 20 percent aerobic work intervals. Thus much of your training will use the distances over which you would normally race—as you might expect—but you should also include some workouts with longer distances, such as the 220- and even the 440-yard swims. If you are a long-distance swimmer, most of your workouts will of course be over the longer distances, with only a few shorter anaerobic workouts.

For the serious competitive swimmer, building your cardiovascular capacity by running is not very effective for swimming. That's because swimming calls for different muscle mechanics and special skills, so you ought to follow swimming I.T. programs exclusively. If your swimming workouts are restricted, however, you can supplement your workouts with weight training, particularly on the type of machines that simulates swimming stroke movements. Weight training is especially useful for divers. Divers can also incorporate trampoline work and bench stepping to develop leg power. We'll have more to say about such exercises in later chapters.

Swimmers, of course, should not limit themselves to the three-times-a-week workout of the nonathlete. Most swimmers find it necessary to work out every day or even twice a day. Whether you work out once a day or more often is up to you and your coach. What is important is that you work out intervally for maximum benefit from your program.

Susie Atwood, the Ohio State University head women's swimming coach and former Olympic backstroker, tells us that her varsity team uses a system of interval training which has rest periods of varying lengths. Over the course of the season, Coach Atwood's objective is to decrease the rest times while the repeat swims become faster.

For example, Ms. Atwood says: "At the beginning of the season, I ask the team to do a workout which includes six 400-yard free-style swims in under five minutes and twenty seconds, ten 100-yard kick swims (with a board) in under two minutes, and four 300-yard pulling swims in under four minutes and thirty seconds. After a couple of months, the workout will be the same but the times will be faster by 10 percent and the rest periods are shortened. At least three months of interval training is necessary for the team to reach its peak. Periodically, I ask the girls to check their heart rates, making certain they exceed 160 beats per minute following most sets of swims."

That's a tough program, but it's entirely compatible with the principles of interval training for athletes.

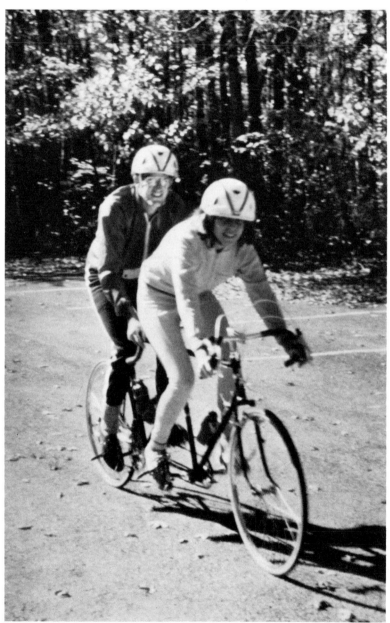

14. Cycling offers a pleasant alternative to running, for interval training—and one that's easier on the feet and ankles.

6 BICYCLING WITH I.T.

Bicycling for General Fitness

Bicycling is an excellent way of improving your general fitness. The benefits to the heart and lungs are comparable to those generated by running, and your leg and stomach muscles will get a fine workout. In fact, some doctors recommend cycling over running because the feet, ankles, legs and back do not suffer the shock of pounding the pavement at every step. And of course, the ordinary bicycle is relatively inexpensive. As a former president of the American Heart Association once said: "We ought to replace the automobile with bicycles. . . . It would be better for our coronaries, our dispositions and certainly our finances."

The bike is also ideally suited to interval training, since you can work hard during your exercise runs and coast or pedal gently during your relief intervals. If you have a bicycle with several gears, you can adjust the resistance to pedaling simply by changing gear: the higher the gear, the greater the resistance to movement (and vice versa). However, if you live in a hilly part of the country, the hills will often provide more than enough resistance.

Bikes are at a disadvantage in wet or icy weather, when the possibility of a skid or a more serious accident is much higher. However, as we've noted before, you can always substitute for your cycling some other activity, such as calisthenics, which can be performed indoors when the weather is bad.

You can also use an exercise bike mounted on a fixed frame and specifically designed for indoor use. Exercise bikes usually have some sort of friction control so you can increase or decrease the resistance of the pedals. Such bikes often have an odometer which measures the distance the exercise bike would have traveled if it were not on a fixed stand. You can use the odometer to measure your distances for interval training too. The exercise bike is very useful for city dwellers, who may not wish to contend with unsympathetic car and truck traffic, to say nothing of the fumes generated thereby.

Arthur Ashe, the professional tennis player, lives in an apartment in Manhattan and, when he's at home, works out daily on his exercise bike, contending that twenty minutes on the bike is more helpful to him as a tennis player than a

15. The stationary bike is eminently suited to interval training because the exercise can be carefully controlled.

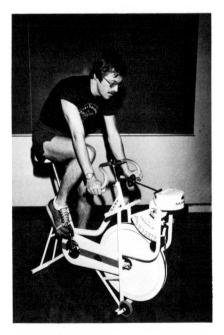

five-mile run. Ashe uses short sprints mixed in with occasional longer "runs" on his bike in a form of interval training that he has found to be the best for him as a tennis player. Tennis players, of course, need to emphasize anaerobic capacity for the fast footwork that's required on the tennis court.

In the San Francisco Bay area, many commuters use bikes to get to the nearest station of the city's rapid transit system, since the bike is far easier to park than an automobile and, naturally, uses no gasoline. If you use a bicycle to commute to school or to your place of work, you can easily adapt your morning and evening runs to an interval training program. That way, you can get your three-times-a-week workout without using much additional time.

In New York City, many parks are closed to vehicular traffic on weekends and evenings during the summer. The parks are ideal for interval training since the bicycle traffic is usually one way and the roads are wide enough to cope with cyclists moving at widely differing speeds. And of course, it's always far more pleasant to cycle in attractive surroundings. You may be able to find parks that allow cycling in your town, too.

Writing Your Own Cycling I.T. Program

You can adapt a running I.T. program for bicycling simply by taking the running distances and multiplying them by a factor of 2½. That's because running one mile is approximately equivalent to cycling two and a half miles in terms of the energy used. So you could take the running programs of Chapter Four and modify them using simple arithmetic. Alternatively, you can start from a table of guidelines as we did in the running and swimming chapters.

You'll see that our chart of guidelines for cycling (Table 18) looks just like the running and swimming charts except that

Guidelines for Writing Your Own Bicycling I.T. Programs

Work Effort	Performance Time	Training Distance (miles)
anaerobic	under 90 seconds	⅛ ¼ ¾
aerobic	over 90 seconds	1¼ 1½ 2

Table 18   The cycling guidelines are very similar to those for running and swimming, except that the distances for the rides are in miles, since they are longer for equivalent effort.

the distances, being rather longer, are given in miles and not yards. We think that you'll find measurements by mile to be more useful, especially if your bicycle has an odometer that measures distance traveled in miles and fractions of a mile.

As we suggested in our earlier chapters, for general conditioning most of your runs should come from the aerobic work effort group, with a few from the anaerobic group. Select your distances and adjust your times on the basis of target heart rates (see Table 4). Naturally, you should take things easy for the first few weeks if you are not a regular bike rider. As an example, your workout on one day of your first week might consist of one 1¼-mile run at an easy pace—"easy" meaning that you do not yet reach your target heart rate—plus eight ¼-mile rides, also at an easy pace. You'll have to time yourself over the rides to determine the proper rest intervals. For the longer ride, your relief interval should be the same time as your ride, while for the shorter ride your relief interval would

Rides Per Workout	Work/Relief Ratio	Type of Relief
24	1:3	rest relief
16	1:3	rest relief
8	1:2	work relief
4	1:1	work relief
3	2:1	rest relief
3	2:1	rest relief

be three times as long as the time taken to complete the ride.

As your program progresses, you should shorten the time for your rides to keep within your target heart rates for both work and relief intervals. At the end of an eight-week I.T. program, a healthy twenty-year-old might have a workout of one 2-mile ride and two 1½-mile rides on one day with, say, sixteen ¼-mile rides on another day. Such workouts will help increase the capacity of both the aerobic and anaerobic systems.

If you'd rather not work out your own specific I.T. program, we have some suggestions for cycling I.T. programs for various age groups (see Tables 19–21). However, we must emphasize, once again, that these are merely suggestions. By all means try our programs, but be ready to modify them according to your heart-rate response if they are too hard or too easy for you. Using the table of guidelines, you can alter our programs to customize them for you.

Bicycling I.T. Program for Under 30s

Week	Day	Rides	Distance (miles)	Time (minutes: seconds)	Relief Interval (minutes: seconds)
1	1	4	¼	easy*	1:3*
		8	⅛	easy	1:3
	2	2	¾	easy	1:3
		8	⅛	easy	1:3
	3	1	1¼	easy	1:3
		6	¼	easy	1:3
2	1	2	1¼	easy	1:3
		2	¾	easy	1:3
	2	6	1¼	easy	1:3
	3	1	4	easy	—
3	1	2	1	3:00	6:00
		2	¾	2:15	4:30
	2	12	¼	0:45	2:15
	3	1	1¼	3:45	3:45
		2	¾	2:15	4:30
4	1	3	1	2:55	5:50
		3	¾	2:15	4:30
	2	16	¼	0:45	2:15
	3	2	1¼	3:40	3:40
		2	¾	2:15	4:30
5	1	4	1	2:50	5:40
		2	¾	2:15	4:30
	2	16	¼	0:40	2:00
	3	2	1¼	3:40	3:40
		2	¾	2:15	4:30
6	1	4	1	2:45	5:30
		2	¾	2:13	4:26
	2	16	¼	0:39	1:57
	3	2	1¼	3:35	3:35
		2	¾	2:13	4:26
7	1	2	1¼	3:30	3:30
		2	¾	2:10	4:20
	2	16	¼	0:38	1:54
	3	1	2	5:30	2:45
		2	1½	4:05	2:02
8	1	2	1¼	3:25	3:25
		2	¾	2:10	4:20
	2	16	¼	0:36	1:48
	3	1	2	5:25	2:42
		2	1½	4:00	2:00

Table 19
    *For rides at an "easy" pace, the relief interval should be three times as long as the time taken to complete one ride.

Bicycling I.T. Program for 30s–50s

Week	Day	Rides	Distance (miles)	Time (minutes: seconds)	Relief Interval (minutes: seconds)
1	1	4	¼	easy*	1:3*
		8	⅛	easy	1:3
	2	2	¾	easy	1:3
		8	⅛	easy	1:3
	3	1	1¼	easy	1:3
		6	¼	easy	1:3
2	1	2	1¼	easy	1:3
		2	¾	easy	1:3
	2	6	1¼	easy	1:3
	3	1	4	easy	—
3	1	2	1	3:45	7:30
		2	¾	2:45	5:30
	2	12	¼·	0:50	2:30
	3	1	1¼	4:40	4:40
		2	¾	2:45	5:30
4	1	3	1	3:40	7:20
		3	¾	2:45	5:30
	2	16	¼	0:50	2:30
	3	2	1¼	4:35	4:35
		2	¾	2:45	5:30
5	1	4	1	3:35	7:10
		2	¾	2:45	5:30
	2	16	¼	0:48	2:24
	3	2	1¼	4:30	4:30
		2	¾	2:45	5:30
6	1	4	1	3:30	7:00
		2	¾	2:40	5:20
	2	16	¼	0:48	2:24
	3	2	1¼	4:25	4:25
		2	¾	2:40	5:20
7	1	2	1¼	4:20	4:20
		2	¾	2:40	5:20
	2	16	¼	0:45	2:15
	3	1	2	6:20	3:10
		2	1½	5:00	2:30
8	1	2	1¼	4:20	4:20
		2	¾	2:35	5:10
	2	16	¼	0:45	2:15
	3	1	2	6:10	3:05
		2	1½	4:50	2:25

Table 20
*For rides at an "easy" pace, the relief interval should be three times as long as the time taken to complete one ride.

Bicycling I.T. Program for Over 50s

Week	Day	Rides	Distance (miles)	Time (minutes: seconds)	Relief Interval (minutes: seconds)
1	1	4	¼	easy*	1:3*
		8	⅛	easy	1:3
	2	2	¾	easy	1:3
		8	⅛	easy	1:3
	3	1	1¼	easy	1:3
		6	¼	easy	1:3
2	1	2	1¼	easy	1:3
		2	¾	easy	1:3
	2	6	1¼	easy	1:3
	3	1	4	easy	—
3	1	2	1	4:40	9:20
			¾	3:25	6:50
	2	12	¼	1:00	3:00
	3	1	1¼	5:50	5:50
		2	¾	3:25	6:50
4	1	3	1	4:35	9:10
		3	¾	3:25	6:50
	2	16	¼	1:00	3:00
	3	2	1¼	5:45	5:45
		2	¾	3:25	6:50
5	1	4	1	4:30	9:00
		2	¾	3:25	6:50
	2	16	¼	0:58	2:54
	3	2	1¼	5:40	5:40
		2	¾	3:25	6:50
6	1	4	1	4:25	8:50
		2	¾	3:20	6:40
	2	16	¼	0:58	2:54
	3	2	1¼	5:35	5:35
		2	¾	3:20	6:40
7	1	2	1¼	5:30	5:30
		2	¾	3:20	6:40
	2	16	¼	0:55	2:45
	3	1	2	7:30	3:45
		2	1½	6:15	3:07
8	1	2	1¼	5:25	5:25
		2	¾	3:15	6:30
	2	16	¼	0:55	2:45
	3	1	2	7:20	3:40
		2	1½	6:10	3:05

Table 21

*For rides at an "easy" pace, the relief interval should be three times as long as the time taken to complete one ride.

How to Use the Bicycling I.T. Tables

Our cycling I.T. programs are designed the same way as our running and swimming programs. There are three workouts per week for an eight-week program to get you in shape. At the end of the eight-week series, two workouts per week should be sufficient to keep you fit. The selection of the two workouts is up to you, but they should be at least as hard as any of the three during the last week of your eight-week program. At the end of the eight-week series you will know which workouts you prefer.

At first, we recommend that you use an "easy" pace that is dependent on your personal condition as you go into the program. Take your pulse frequently during the first couple of weeks so you do not exercise too hard (or too easily). You will note that by the start of the third week, we expect the under-thirty group to be able to reach speeds of around 20 miles per hour for a sufficiently intense workout. If that pace is too stiff for you, exercise at the same distances but make your times a little longer.

For an older first-time cyclist, an easy pace might be as low as 10 miles per hour for the first few workouts. The most important objective is to build your speeds within your capacity without undue strain on your heart and lungs during the first few weeks. It's best, too, to start your I.T. workouts on a level track or stretch of road: you'll make things too easy if you're going downhill and too tough if you have to struggle uphill.

You'll see that the tables suggest a relief interval that's three times as long as the time to complete a ride for the workouts in the first couple of weeks. If you take five minutes to do a 1-mile ride, you should then rest for fifteen minutes. For the third and subsequent weeks, the tables give you times for each run and for the relief intervals to use between each run. For example, for the under-thirty group, the first workout of the third week should be two 1-mile rides at three minutes, with a six-minute relief interval after each ride, plus two ¾-mile rides in two minutes and fifteen seconds, with a relief interval of four minutes and thirty seconds after each ride.

Don't forget to check your heart rate occasionally during your workouts. It's important that you reach the proper target heart rate for your age group (see Table 4), but it's also important that you don't do too much. If your heart does not recover as quickly as it should during your relief intervals, wait a little longer before you exercise again. If your heart rate does not appear to recover during the relief intervals, stop for the rest of the day. Any signs of a continuing problem with high heart rates are an indication you should seek professional advice from your physician. Remember, do not ignore those early warning signals from your body.

Combining Cycling with Other I.T. Programs

In Chapter Five, we mentioned the suburban couple who bike and swim before commuting to work. You can easily combine cycling with other exercises in an I.T. program. By now you will have recognized the similarity between our guideline tables for various activities. It will be obvious that you can substitute one activity for another at the same level of the table.

For example, cycling 1¼ miles is approximately equivalent to running 880 yards or swimming 220 yards. So if your program calls for a 1¼-mile bike ride, you can do an 880-yard run in about the same time if you wish. You'll remember we said that cycling distances are about two and a half times the running distances, and that swimming distances are one fourth the running distances (or one tenth the cycling distances, if you prefer to mix swimming and biking). It's an easy matter to make the conversions from one program to another.

Remember, though, that a sudden switch from, say, cycling to running will probably slow your times somewhat. You may have to allow a little extra time until your body gets used to the new form of exercise.

You can also combine calisthenics and weight training with cycling by using comparable performance times. For example, a 1¼-mile bike run in three minutes is equivalent to forty two-count exercises, also completed in three minutes. It's a little more difficult to develop a suitable mix of calisthenics with running, swimming or cycling, but you can do it by comparing the appropriate tables of guidelines. If you wish to add calisthenics to your I.T. program, you may have to experiment a little to find the right mix for you. However, all our I.T. programs are completely flexible. Your own I.T. program is individual to you and should be written by you.

Training for Cycling Events

Competitive cycling has long been a relatively popular sport in Europe at both the professional and the amateur levels. It is just now gaining momentum here in the U.S. Virtually all the top road racers use some form of interval training for both their road work and their off-the-road conditioning. Many cyclists combine weight training, to develop the muscles used in cycling, with sprints and longer rides, to increase the capacity of the heart and lungs.

You can develop an I.T. program of cycling and weight training for competitive cycling using the guidelines in this book. As an athlete, you will probably wish to work out on a daily basis and to use longer distances than we have suggested in our guidelines. Your program should concentrate on the distances at which you intend to compete, but we do

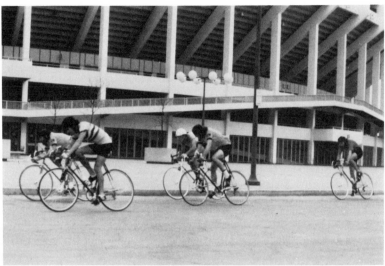

16. Racing cyclists should use interval training to prepare for their events.

feel you should mix in some shorter distances even if you are a long-distance road racer. Although road racing is often an aerobic activity, most races call for sudden sprints which make extreme demands on your anaerobic energy systems. Your training program should improve the development of all your energy systems. If you intend to compete in short-distance sprint events, naturally your training will concentrate more on the anaerobic distances, with only a few longer aerobic runs added in. The exact form of your I.T. program is up to you.

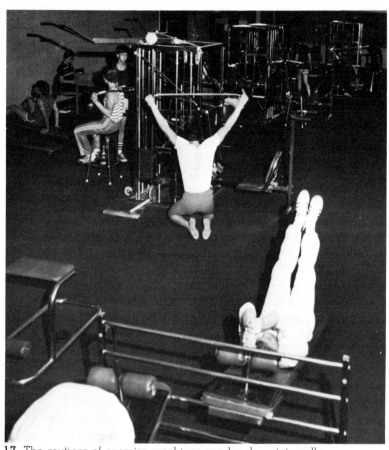

17. The routines of exercise machines can be done intervally.

7 CALISTHENICS, WEIGHT TRAINING AND BENCH STEPPING WITH I.T.

Calisthenics and Weight Training for General Fitness

As we noted in an earlier chapter, running is often the easiest way for the average person to get physically fit and stay that way. However, you can also use calisthenics, weight lifting or bench stepping to train intervally, although such programs are a little more complicated to design than a simple running, swimming, or bicycling I.T. program. You'll remember, of course, that we suggested a number of calisthenic exercises for your warm-up sessions before getting into your workout proper. You can use any of those exercises for a calisthenic I.T. program or you can use groups of exercises from other exercise programs. In fact, the selection of the exercises is probably one of the more difficult parts of devising a calisthenic I.T. program, because the choice is so open.

If you do use a variety of exercises in your workouts, you'll be able to strengthen a wider range of muscle groups than those used in running. While running is excellent for the leg muscles and some stomach muscles, the upper body is little used, even if you do pump your arms vigorously as you run. By contrast, using only two exercises, such as push-ups and squat jumps, will exercise most of the major muscle groups of your body. So calisthenics are a very acceptable alternative to running, swimming, or biking as the basis of an interval training program.

There's another quite significant advantage to calisthenics and bench stepping: you can often do the exercises at home without special equipment. All you'll need is a room with enough space for you to move around as you exercise. And of course, your workouts will not be affected by the weather outside, although we do suggest that you do not exercise, indoors or out, on very hot and humid days or when the level of air pollution is high. Weight lifting does require special equipment and should be done under supervision.

Writing Your Own Calisthenic
and Weight Training I.T. Programs

Up to this point, we've looked at I.T. programs that are based on training distances for either running, or swimming or bicycling. However, you'll probably remember that our tables of guidelines for writing your own I.T. programs were divided into anaerobic and aerobic effort areas, based on the time of a particular run, swim or bike ride. Our guidelines for calisthenics and weight training are based on the same times. We need only to construct programs with specific numbers of exercises to be completed in various time periods.

Let's take a brief example: Part of a running program might call for you to run two 880s in three minutes—an aerobic exercise, for the most part. Let's say that we wish to replace this run with squat jumps (jumping straight up in the air from a crouched position and then returning to the crouch). By experimenting for yourself, you might determine that you could do 45 squat jumps in three minutes, so your workout might consist of two sets of 45 squat jumps, each set done in three minutes (with an appropriate rest interval between the two sets, of course).

Fortunately, we do not have to go through that kind of conversion to set up a calisthenic I.T. program. Instead, we can start from a table of guidelines based on training times, instead of on training distances as in the earlier chapters. You'll see that Table 22 is divided into anaerobic and aerobic effort areas, as was the case for the running, swimming, and biking programs. But now we list the performance time for each group of exercises from ten seconds to five minutes. We can now write our own calisthenic or weight lifting plans just as we did for the running, swimming, and biking programs.

For example, let's say you can do ten toe touches in 25 seconds. A workout consisting entirely of toe touches might have 25 repetitions of ten toe touches, each group done in twenty seconds with one-minute rest intervals. Alternatively, you might want to add a second exercise, say, sit-ups, and to do those aerobically. Thus your program might consist of ten repetitions of ten toe touches plus four repetitions of 25 sit-ups. Of course, you can use as many different exercises as you wish. It's just a matter of determining how many you should do in a certain time period for various proportions of aerobic or anaerobic effort.

As with the running, swimming, and biking programs, we suggest you begin very slowly for the first couple of weeks. Check your heart rate frequently and adjust the number of exercises and the rate of performance to keep your heart rate on target (see Table 4). As your fitness improves, you will have to make your workouts harder.

For general fitness, we think that 70 percent of your workout should concentrate on aerobic exercises and 30 percent on anaerobic exercises. Quite obviously, exercises that you can do very rapidly will lend themselves to anaerobic per-

Guidelines for Writing Your Own Calisthenic and Weight

Work Effort	Training Time	Repetitions Per Workout
anaerobic	under 10 seconds	50
	10–30 seconds	25
	30–90 seconds	10
aerobic	1½–2 minutes	8
	2–3 minutes	5
	3–5 minutes	3

Table 22   This table shows how many repetitions of a group of exercises should be done in one workout. If you can do 5 toe touches in under 10 seconds, 50 sets of 10 toe touches might comprise one workout (for anaerobic conditioning).

formance and longer ones to aerobic performance. Since writing a calisthenic I.T. program is more challenging than a simple running, swimming or bicycling plan, you might like to start with our suggested I.T. programs (see tables 23–25) and then modify those programs to suit your own purposes.

If you'd prefer to devise your own program, you may find rates of exercising easier to work out if you use a simple rule of thumb instead of experimenting and checking yourself by measuring your heart rate. The rule is to allow one second for each count of the exercise for anaerobic effort and two seconds per count for aerobic effort. The count is just the rhythm of the exercise. For example, sit-ups are a two-count exercise —up on "one" and down again on "two." Thus we would say that a sit-up is a two-count exercise.

If you wish to do sit-ups anaerobically, allow two seconds for each sit-up (i.e., twenty seconds for ten sit-ups). Should you decide to do sit-ups aerobically, you would allow four se-

Training I.T. Programs	
Work/Relief Ratio	Type of Relief
1:3	rest relief
1:3	rest relief
1:3	work relief
1:2	work relief
1:1	rest relief
2:1	rest relief

conds for each one (i.e., forty seconds for ten sit-ups). This will give you a good base from which to start if you are reasonably fit. However, if you are beginning an exercise program for the first time, you might double those times until you get well into your routine.

Of course, you will want to speed up your rate of exercising as your program progresses. Our numbers are simply suggestions. Only you can determine how fast you should exercise and how fast you should move along from week to week.

How to Use the Calisthenic and Weight Training I.T. Tables
Since calisthenic and weight lifting exercises can be performed in a variety of ways, we've suggested two sets of I.T. programs for each of our age groupings. The tables are for exercises that can be done to a two-count rhythm, such as

A four-count calisthenic exercise. The squat thrust is an excellent four-count exercise for a calisthenic I.T. program. From a standing position, take a deep knee bend, placing your hands on the floor in front of you in a resting position (count "one"). Jump and extend your legs backward to a front-leaning position with your body supported by your hands and toes (count "two"). Return to the squat-rest position (count "three"). Stand up with your arms by your sides and your head up (count "four").

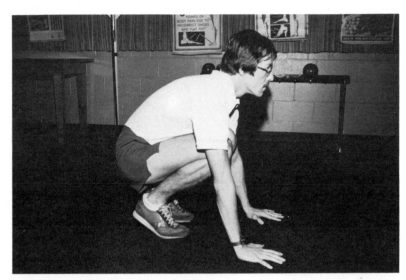

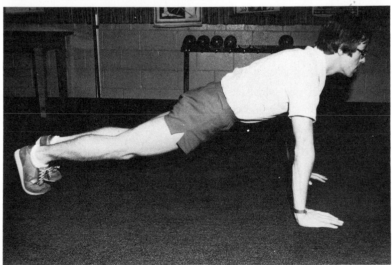

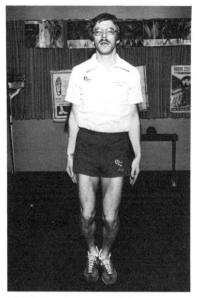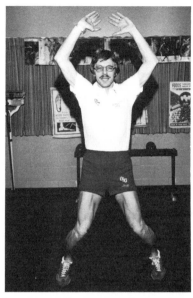

19. A two-count calisthenic exercise: Jumping jacks are an effective two-count exercise for a calisthenic I.T. program. From a standing position with your arms by your side (*above, left*), jump up in the air, spreading your legs apart and (*above, right*) bringing your arms up over your head (count "one"). Return to the starting position for a count of "two."

squat jumps, but they can be used for exercises that may be done to a four-count rhythm, such as squat thrusts, by dividing the number of exercises by two. The selection of the actual exercises is up to you. It's best to use several exercises, but you'll find the going easier if they are all of the same count so you can stick to one program, especially in the first few weeks.

Let's suppose that you wish to do sit-ups and arm raises for your workouts. If you are under thirty (see Table 23), on the first day of the first week you might attempt four sets of fifteen sit-ups, the fifteen to be done in forty seconds with a two-minute rest interval between work periods. You could then follow this with, say, eight sets of eight arm raises, each group of eight to be done in twenty seconds with a one-minute rest

Calisthenics and Weight Training I.T. Program for Under 30s
(Two-count exercises)*

Week	Day	Repetitions	Number of Exercises	Time for One Repetition (minutes: seconds)	Relief Interval (minutes: seconds)
1	1	4	15	0:40	2:00
		8	8	0:20	1:00
	2	2	50	1:20	2:40
		8	8	0:20	1:00
	3	1	40	3:00	3:00
		6	15	0:40	2:00
2	1	2	40	3:00	3:00
		2	50	1:20	2:40
	2	6	50	1:20	2:40
	3	1	75	5:00	—
3	1	3	36	2:20	4:40
		3	40	1:20	2:40
	2	15	20	0:40	2:00
	3	2	50	3:00	3:00
		3	40	1:20	2:40
4	1	6	36	2:20	4:40
	2	20	20	0:40	2:00
	3	2	50	3:00	3:00
		5	40	1:20	2:40
5	1	3	40	2:20	4:40
		5	45	1:20	2:40
	2	20	25	0:40	2:00
	3	2	60	3:00	3:00
		5	45	1:20	2:40
6	1	3	50	2:20	4:40
		5	50	1:20	2:40
	2	20	30	0:40	2:00
	3	2	70	3:00	3:00
		5	50	1:20	2:40
7	1	2	80	3:00	3:00
		5	55	1:20	2:40
	2	20	35	1:20	2:40
	3	2	100	4:30	4:30
		2	80	3:00	3:00
8	1	2	90	3:00	3:00
		5	60	1:20	2:40
	2	20	40	0:40	2:00
	3	2	110	4:30	4:30
		2	90	3:00	3:00

Table 23
*Divide number of exercises by two for four-count exercises.

Calisthenics and Weight Training I.T. Program for 30s–50s
(Two-count exercises)*

Week	Day	Repetitions	Number of Exercises	Time for One Repetition (minutes: seconds)	Relief Interval (minutes: seconds)
1	1	4	10	0:40	2:00
		8	5	0:20	1:00
	2	2	35	1:20	2:40
		8	5	0:20	1:00
	3	1	30	3:00	3:00
		6	10	0:40	2:00
2	1	2	30	3:00	3:00
		2	40	1:20	2:40
	2	6	40	1:20	2:40
	3	1	55	5:00	—
3	1	3	25	2:20	4:40
		3	30	1:20	2:40
	2	15	15	0:40	2:00
	3	2	40	3:00	3:00
		3	30	1:20	2:40
4	1	6	25	2:20	4:40
	2	20	15	0:40	2:00
	3	2	40	3:00	3:00
		5	30	1:20	2:40
5	1	3	30	2:20	4:40
		5	35	1:20	2:40
	2	20	20	0:40	2:00
	3	2	45	3:00	3:00
		5	35	1:20	2:40
6	1	3	40	2:20	4:40
		5	40	1:20	2:40
	2	20	20	0:40	2:00
	3	2	55	3:00	3:00
		5	40	1:20	2:40
7	1	2	60	3:00	3:00
		5	45	1:20	2:40
	2	20	25	0:40	2:00
	3	2	75	4:30	4:30
		2	60	3:00	3:00
8	1	2	65	3:00	3:00
		5	45	1:20	2:40
	2	20	30	0:40	2:00
	3	2	85	4:30	4:30
		2	65	3:00	3:00

Table 24
*Divide number of exercises by two for four-count exercises.

Calisthenics and Weight Training I.T. Program for Over 50s
(Two-count exercises)*

Week	Day	Repetitions	Number of Exercises	Time for One Repetition (minutes: seconds)	Relief Interval (minutes: seconds)
1	1	4	8	0:40	2:00
		8	3	0:20	1:00
	2	2	30	1:20	2:40
		8	3	0:20	1:00
	3	1	25	3:00	3:00
		6	8	0:40	2:00
2	1	2	25	3:00	3:00
		2	35	1:20	2:40
	2	6	35	1:20	2:40
	3	1	50	5:00	---
3	1	3	20	2:20	4:40
		3	25	1:20	2:40
	2	15	10	0:40	2:00
	3	2	35	3:00	3:00
		3	25	1:20	2:40
4	1	6	20	2:20	4:40
	2	20	10	0:40	2:00
	3	2	35	3:00	3:00
		5	25	1:20	2:40
5	1	3	25	2:20	4:40
		5	30	1:20	2:40
	2	20	15	0:40	2:00
	3	2	40	3:00	3:00
		5	30	1:20	2:40
6	1	3	35	2:20	4:40
		5	35	1:20	2:40
	2	20	15	0:40	2:00
	3	2	50	3:00	3:00
		5	35	1:20	2:40
7	2	20	20	0:40	2:00
	3	2	60	4:30	4:30
		2	55	3:00	3:00
8	1	2	60	3:00	3:00
		5	40	1:20	2:40
	2	20	25	0:40	2:00
	3	2	75	4:30	4:30
		2	60	3:00	3:00

Table 25
*Divide number of exercises by two for four-count exercises.

period between each work interval. Alternatively, you could reverse the order and do four sets of fifteen arm raises, followed by eight sets of eight sit-ups.

Provided that your exercises are of the two-count variety, you can mix them up in any way you choose. This type of I.T. program is well suited to the exercises of Chapter Three or to the kinds of exercise found in the RCAF fitness books. The selection of the exercises is up to you and the mix that you use in your workout is also at your discretion. In fact, you can vary the exercises from day to day and week to week.

If you wish to use four-count exercises, simply halve the number of exercises in the workout or portion of the workout. For example, you could do four sets of fifteen sit-ups, as in the previous example, and then substitute eight sets of four squat thrusts for the arm raises. So you can devise workouts that consist of two-count exercises, four-count exercises or any combination of the types of exercise.

Don't be tempted to cut the exercises short so you can get them done in the time suggested. Each count should be done over the full range of motion whenever possible. This will ensure that you get the most from the exercise in terms of improving both your muscular strength and your flexibility. If you cannot do the number of exercises suggested in the time recommended, don't worry. Just do as many as you can. You'll see from the tables that the times remain pretty constant from week to week, but the number of repetitions increases. If you start with a smaller number of repetitions, you can increase the number each week by a corresponding amount—but don't try to catch up. It's best to stretch out your training program if the work rates are too stiff for you at first.

Of course, the opposite can happen too. You may find you can easily do the number of exercises in the time suggested. If that's the case, you can either increase the number of exercises to be done within the work interval or you can increase the difficulty of the exercise. As an example of the latter, you might do your sit-ups on an inclined board or your arm raises using light weights. However, be extremely careful about increasing the intensity of the exercises too soon and too much. We suggest you wait until the fifth week before modifying your exercises to make them harder.

It's all too easy to develop excessively sore muscles when you are unused to regular calisthenics. Give your muscles time to get used to the exercises before you tax them too hard. If extreme muscular soreness is a problem, you may be doing too much. Ease off for a few days until the muscles recover. Continuing to exercise with overly sore muscles is a sure way

20. A four-count weight training exercise: The arm raise with light dumbells can be done as a four-count exercise. Start with the dumbbells hanging by your side (*below, left*), raise them outward so your arms are horizontal (count "one"), then raise them further so your arms make a "V" (count "two") and finally (*below, right*) with your arms stretched above your head (count "three"). Bring your arms back to the starting position for the final count ("four").

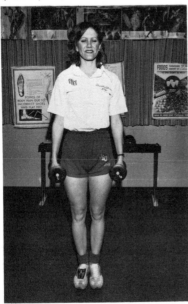
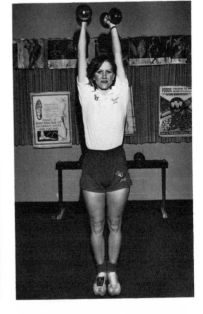

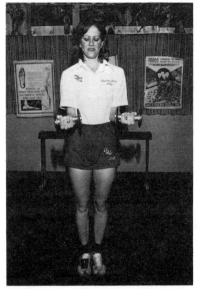 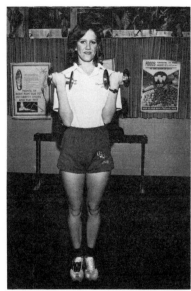

21. A two-count weight training exercise: Wrist curls with light dumbbells are a good two-count exercise. Start with the dumbbells held out in front of you (*above, left*) and raise them to your shoulders (*above, right*) for a count of "one." Return the weights to the starting position for a count of "two."

to do some more serious damage. Remember that a sore muscle is a message to you. Ignore the message and you may hurt your body. As we've stressed before, you are the one who knows your body best: you must be the one who listens to its early warning signals.

Bench Stepping I. T. Programs

Bench stepping can be done almost anywhere at any time by anyone. The exercise lends itself very well to interval training. Bench stepping does not need expensive equipment, needs little area in which to exercise, requires little skill, is easy to regulate in terms of exercise intensity and can be done by people with no previous exercise experience.

You can change the intensity of bench stepping by altering the height of the bench or by changing the stepping frequency. To simplify the exercises, we've used a fixed bench height of 16 inches for our suggested interval training programs, so you'll see that the stepping rate is the only item to change as you progress.

For bench stepping, you'll need a sturdy bench that's very stable. You can build a 16-inch-high bench from plywood or particle board (see photograph) or you can use two steps of a normal staircase (most stairs have an eight-inch riser from

22. You can build a sturdy bench for bench stepping at home or in the office but almost any strong bench will do.

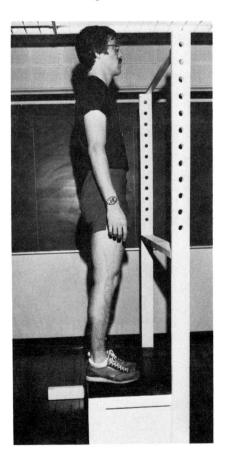

step to step). Don't use a chair: most chairs are at least 18 inches high and are neither strong nor stable enough to permit repeated stepping.

The only difficulty you may run into with bench stepping is developing the proper cadence for your exercises. The best way, we've found, is to use a musician's metronome, setting the dial to four times the desired pace. For example, if you wish to exercise at the rate of thirty steps per minute, the metronome is set at 120 clicks per minute. With each four clicks, say to yourself: "Up, Up, Down, Down." In other words, step up first with one foot and then with the other. Then step down with the first foot, followed by the other. This way, you will do thirty complete steps in one minute.

If you do not have a metronome, a large clock with a sweep-second hand will help you to keep the proper cadence. For a bench stepping program we devised for the U.S. Navy submarine squadrons, the cadence was put on a tape cassette as a series of voice commands. The entire program, including the rest intervals, was on three cassettes. This had the advantage of allowing the program to be played over the public address system so the entire crew could exercise at the same time. Of course, this kind of sophistication isn't really necessary for individual exercise.

Bench stepping is an excellent activity for people who are cooped up all day in an office. A few years ago, a dentist called one of us seeking advice on exercise. He prefaced his request by stating that he flatly refused to jog or even walk outdoors. "I'd rather die," he said, "than be chased by dogs, harassed by cars or be exposed to inclement weather." We recommended bench stepping for this unintrepid dentist since it's a form of exercise he can do indoors, perhaps in his office between patients. He recorded his program on a cassette tape and built his own bench. So far as we know, he is still bench stepping intervally.

For the bench stepping programs, the relief interval should consist of walking in place, moderately flexing the arms and legs, or stepping back and forth (about 18 inches) on the floor level at the same frequency as during the work interval.

How To Use the Bench Stepping I.T. Tables

Although our bench stepping I.T. programs are designed in the same way as the running, swimming and bicycling programs, the tables are a little different. That's largely because we've added a column listing the cadence—the number of steps per minute—for each work interval. This will help you if you're using a metronome to pace your bench stepping.

For example, during the first week of the program for under-30's, the first day should consist of a workout of two sets of work intervals. The first set has four intervals where you step on and off the bench 18 times in 40 seconds. This corresponds to a stepping rate of 27 times a minute. After each 18 steps, rest or walk slowly for two minutes. After those four work intervals (and their associated relief intervals), the second half of the workout asks you to do eight intervals of nine steps in 20 seconds with a one-minute relief interval between each work interval. That also corresponds to a rate of 27 steps per minute so there's no need to reset your metronome between the two halves of the workout.

As the weeks progress, you'll see that the rate of stepping is increased to a maximum of 36 steps per minute. At the same time, the number of steps is increased and the rest intervals become shorter. Thus, the program becomes progressively tougher in keeping with the principles of interval training. At the end of the eight weeks, you'll be able to keep fit with only one workout per week. You should use the workout listed for the first day of the eighth week. That will give you a sufficient amount of exercise to stay at peak fitness.

Bench Stepping I.T. Program for Under 30s

Week	Day	Number of Work Intervals	Cadence (steps/minute)	Steps/Interval	Time for One Interval (minutes:seconds)	Relief Interval (minutes:seconds)
1	1	4	27	18	0:40	2:00
		8	27	9	0:20	1:00
	2	2	27	36	1:20	2:40
		8	27	9	0:20	1:00
	3	1	27	81	3:00	3:00
		6	27	18	0:40	2:00
2	1	2	27	81	3:00	3:00
		2	27	36	1:20	2:40
	2	6	27	36	1:20	2:40
	3	1	27	135	5:00	—
3	1	15	30	20	0:40	2:00
	2	2	30	90	3:00	3:00
		3	30	40	1:20	2:40
	3	3	30	70	2:20	4:40
		3	30	40	1:20	2:40
4	1	6	33	77	2:20	4:40
	2	20	33	22	0:40	2:00
	3	2	33	99	3:00	3:00
		5	33	44	1:20	2:40
5	1	3	36	84	2:20	4:40
		5	36	48	1:20	2:40
	2	20	36	24	0:40	2:00
	3	2	36	108	3:00	3:00
		5	36	48	1:20	2:40
6	1	3	36	84	2:20	2:20
		5	36	48	1:20	1:20
	2	20	36	20	0:40	1:00
	3	3	36	108	3:00	1:30
		5	36	48	1:20	1:20
7	1	2	36	117	3:00	1:30
		5	36	52	1:20	0:40
	2	20	36	26	0:40	0:40
	3	2	36	175	4:30	2:15
		2	36	117	3:00	1:30
8	1	2	36	117	3:00	1:30
		5	36	52	1:20	0:40
	2	20	36	26	0:40	0:40
	3	2	36	175	4:30	2:15
		2	36	117	3:00	1:30

Table 26

Bench Stepping I.T. Program for 30s–50s

Week	Day	Number of Work Intervals	Cadence (steps/minute)	Steps/Interval	Time for One Interval (minutes: seconds)	Relief Interval (minutes: seconds)
1	1	4	24	16	0:40	2:00
		6	24	8	0:20	1:00
	2	2	24	32	1:20	2:40
		6	24	8	0:20	1:00
	3	1	24	72	3:00	3:00
		4	24	16	0:40	2:00
2	1	2	24	72	3:00	3:00
		2	24	32	1:20	2:40
	2	6	24	32	1:20	2:40
	3	1	24	120	5:00	—
3	1	12	27	18	0:40	2:00
	2	2	27	81	3:00	3:00
		2	27	36	1:20	2:40
	3	3	27	63	2:20	4:40
		3	27	36	1:20	2:40
4	1	6	27	63	2:20	4:40
	2	15	27	18	0:40	2:00
	3	2	27	81	3:00	3:00
		4	27	36	1:20	2:40
5	1	15	30	20	0:40	2:00
	2	2	30	90	3:00	3:00
		4	30	40	1:20	2:40
	3	2	30	70	2:20	4:40
		5	30	40	1:20	2:40
6	1	3	33	77	2:20	2:20
		5	33	44	1:20	1:20
	2	15	33	22	0:40	1:00
	3	3	33	99	3:00	1:30
		5	33	44	1:20	1:20
7	1	2	36	72	3:00	1:30
		4	36	48	1:20	1:20
	2	15	36	24	0:40	1:00
	3	1	36	162	4:30	2:15
		2	36	72	3:00	1:30
8	1	2	36	72	3:00	1:30
		5	36	48	1:20	1:20
	2	15	36	24	0:40	1:00
	3	2	36	162	4:30	2:15
		2	36	72	3:00	1:30

Table 27

Bench Stepping I.T. Program for Over 50s

Week	Day	Number of Work Intervals	Cadence (steps/ minute)	Steps/ Interval	Time for One Interval (minutes: seconds)	Relief Interval (minutes: seconds)
1	1	4	18	12	0:40	2:00
		5	18	6	0:20	1:00
	2	2	18	24	1:20	2:40
		5	18	6	0:20	1:00
	3	1	18	54	3:00	3:00
		3	18	12	0:40	2:00
2	1	2	18	54	3:00	3:00
		2	18	24	1:20	2:40
	2	6	18	24	1:20	2:40
	3	1	18	90	5:00	—
3	1	10	21	14	0:40	2:00
	2	2	21	63	3:00	3:00
		2	21	28	1:20	2:40
	3	3	21	49	2:20	4:40
		3	21	28	1:20	2:40
4	1	6	21	49	2:20	4:40
	2	12	21	14	0:40	2:00
	3	2	21	63	3:00	3:00
		4	21	28	1:20	2:40
5	1	12	24	16	0:40	2:00
	2	2	24	72	3:00	3:00
		4	24	32	1:20	2:40
	3	2	24	56	2:20	4:40
		4	24	32	1:20	2:40
6	1	3	24	56	2:20	2:20
		4	24	32	1:20	1:20
	2	15	24	16	0:40	1:00
	3	3	24	72	3:00	1:30
		4	24	32	1:20	1:20
7	1	2	27	81	3:00	1:30
		3	27	36	1:20	1:20
	2	15	27	18	0:40	1:00
	3	1	27	121	4:30	2:15
		2	27	81	3:00	1:30
8	1	2	27	81	3:00	1:30
		4	27	36	1:20	1:20
	2	15	27	18	0:40	1:00
	3	2	27	121	4:30	2:15
		2	27	81	3:00	1:30

Table 28

Combining Calisthenics with Other I.T. Programs

Although the guidelines for formulating your own I.T. programs for running, swimming, and bicycling look different from the calisthenics guidelines, the basis for constructing the tables is the same. So you can combine calisthenics with running, swimming or bicycling in any way you wish. You could even devise an I.T. program that includes all four activities.

For example, you might divide our suggested programs into three parts, taking one third of the running workouts, one third of the swimming workouts, and one third of the calisthenic workouts. Typically, a day's workout might consist of, say, a couple of 110-yard runs, a couple of 25-yard swims, plus two repetitions of 36 sit-ups, all performed at comparable times.

Another alternative, and one that is inherently simpler, might be to use a running workout one day, a swimming workout the next and a calisthenic workout for the third day of the week. So you can see there is complete flexibility in the programs themselves and between the programs. With some experience and a little imagination, you can develop an I.T. program for yourself that is never dull and yet leads you to peak fitness very quickly.

An excellent way of combining calisthenics with jogging is the parcourse circuit or exercise fitness trail, which is a jogging path with marked exercise stations at regular intervals. The parcourse is ideally suited to interval training. A number of communities have parcourse circuits that are open to the public; others are constructed on college and school campuses and can often be used by nonstudents. A number of resorts have set up parcourses as part of their recreational facilities for guests. The Boca Raton Hotel in Florida has a parcourse which winds its way around one of the hotel's golf courses. Often, such facilities are open to the public for a nominal fee. A trip around a parcourse will do you much more good than several rounds of golf.

Ohio State University has a 1¾ mile parcourse within the campus (see illustration below). The course is designed so that those who use it can walk, jog or run, and have the option of stopping off and resting intervally at any of eighteen different exercise stations.

On the course, the exerciser walks between stations 1 and 4, stopping to do light calisthenics: Achilles stretch for ankle flexibility and Achilles tendon loosening, sit-and-reach for hamstring muscles that are most often used in running, toe touches for hamstrings, back, and abdomen, and knee lifts for back muscles and hamstrings.

Exercise stations 5 through 16 tell the exerciser to run between stations. This provides more of a workout for the heart and lungs as the exercises become more vigorous. At stations 5 through 16, the exerciser does jumping jacks to further raise the heart rate and loosen the joints; log hops to improve motor

23. The parcourse fitness circuit begins with an explanation of the principle of exercising, checking your heart rate and resting between exercises. You can easily use a parcourse intervally.

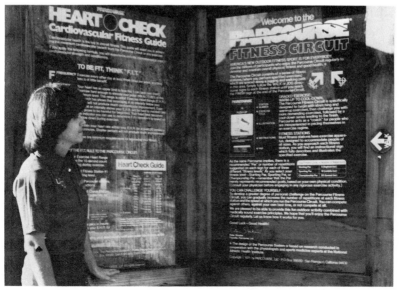

24. A typical parcourse exercise station has a board explaining the exercise (at rear) and some simple equipment for performing the exercise (in this case, a balance beam).

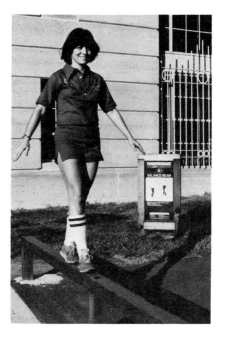

development and coordination and to give a vigorous workout to the calves, thighs, and ankles; the step-up for thighs and knees; the circle body, which is done on a set of rings, for stretching the muscles in the upper body; the body curl for abdominal muscle strengthening and stretching the middle and lower back; chin-ups for strengthening the chest, arms, and shoulders; the hop-kick for the hamstrings, ankles, and calves; the vault bar, to be jumped over while both hands hold the bar; sit-ups for abdominal muscles; push-ups for shoulders and arms; and bench leg raises to further strengthen abdominal muscles.

Stations 15 through 18 are for cooling down and stretching. The exerciser is told to walk between these stations. Exercise station 16 specifies a hand walk for the arms and shoulders, then comes a leg stretch for hip, groin and hamstring muscles, and finally a balance beam for recovery and for improvement

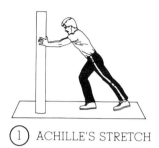

1 ACHILLE'S STRETCH

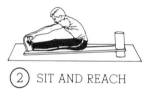

2 SIT AND REACH

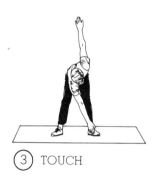

3 TOUCH

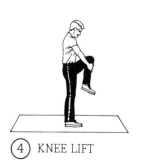

4 KNEE LIFT

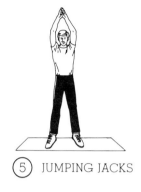

5 JUMPING JACKS

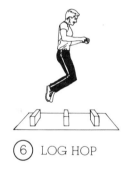

6 LOG HOP

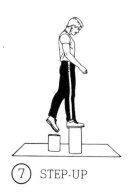

7 STEP-UP

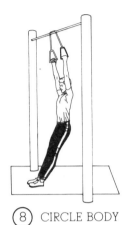

(8) CIRCLE BODY

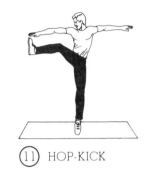

(11) HOP-KICK

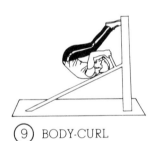

(9) BODY-CURL

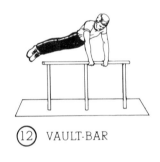

(12) VAULT-BAR

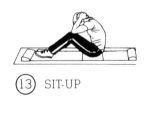

(13) SIT-UP

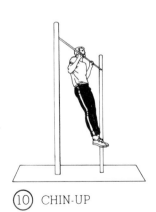

(10) CHIN-UP

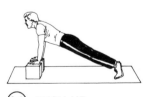

(14) PUSH-UP

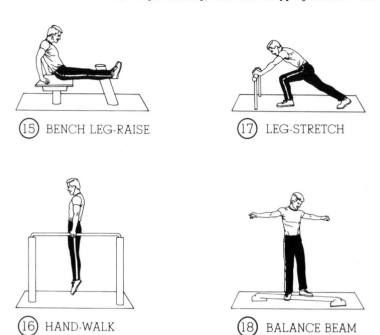

(15) BENCH LEG-RAISE

(17) LEG-STRETCH

(16) HAND-WALK

(18) BALANCE BEAM

of balance and coordination. All the major muscle groups are exercised at least once and the overall progression in the parcourse provides maximum physical activity in a well-coordinated program.

For those who want to achieve a higher level of fitness or who are already in good physical condition, there are four heart check stations to provide a measure of fitness as well as a warning to those who may be pushing too hard. A cardiovascular fitness guide at the beginning of the course explains "pulse-rated" exercise and explains how the participant, by making a ten-second count, can use his or her own heartbeat as a guide to safe and comfortable exercise.

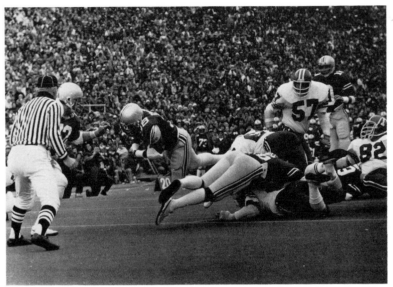

25. Interval training programs can be devised to help any kind of athlete from the weekend sportsman to the professional.

8 PUTTING I.T. TO WORK IN YOUR SPORT

I.T. Can Be Used for Any Sport

By now you've probably realized that interval training is a better way to train athletes for specific sports because I.T. can be used to develop the energy systems that are most heavily used in any particular sport. For example, the football coach who asks his players to run a six-minute mile is not developing the energy sources that are best suited to football. A football player runs at top speed for only a few seconds at a time, and even then, not terribly often. Running a mile in six minutes will not enhance the anaerobic capacity of footballers, but a program of short sprints, done intervally, will do so.

Thus you can see that it is possible to design I.T. programs for athletes from a knowledge of the characteristics of specific sports. However, the needs of athletes will vary considerably depending on the season. During the off season, an athlete should maintain fitness by using an I.T. program of, say, running and weight training. The running workouts should be chosen to increase the capacity of the energy systems needed for the athlete's sport. The weight training exercises could be selected to strengthen the muscles used in that sport, and at the same time would enhance the proper energy systems.

During preseason training, the I.T. programs should become more applicable to the athlete's sport, perhaps including drills that improve the skills needed in that sport. More importantly, the intensity should increase significantly so the athlete arrives close to peak fitness as the season begins.

During the season, of course, most of the training will involve drills that emphasize the skills needed for the sport. However, almost all skill drills can and should be done intervally. An athlete might also wish to continue with a once-a-week workout using the running and weight training program of the preseason training.

By contrast, the weekend athlete can rarely use his or her sport to keep fit in the manner of the high school, college or dedicated amateur athlete. The weekend sportsman should follow an I.T. program similar to that of the athlete's off-season training. A running, swimming, or cycling program might be combined with calisthenics or weight training. The particular plans should be chosen mainly for general conditioning. It's important that the weekend athlete stay fit in order to get the most from the sport and to avoid injuries. Sports such as tennis and golf are pleasant enough social activities but do little for general fitness unless you are fortunate enough to play them every day, as the professionals do. The weekend tennis player or golfer should follow a regular fitness program in addition to engaging in his sport.

Of course, weekend athletes can alter their I.T. programs to emphasize the energy systems of their sports just as regular athletes can. For example, tennis calls for short sprints with fast arm movements and so is mostly an anaerobic sport. Thus the avid tennis player might devise an I.T. program for general conditioning with a bias toward anaerobic workouts.

Off-Season Training for Athletes

Most off-season training programs for the athlete require only that he or she keep moderately active and, perhaps of most concern, keep the body weight at or reasonably near playing weight. With those concerns in mind, we suggest that an off-season training program might consist of some or all of the following:

1. A calisthenic or weight training program that emphasizes increasing strength and power in the muscles the athlete uses for the sport. The specific programs of Chapter Seven could be used or you could write your own program based on our guidelines for various sports (see Table 29).
2. A purely informal (in other words, it's up to you) eight-week I.T. running program of low intensity performed no more than twice a week. The program should be designed

Guidelines for I.T. Sports Programs

Sport	Percent Anaerobic	Percent Aerobic
Badminton	80	20
Baseball	80	20
Basketball	85	15
Cross-country skiing	5	95
Fencing	90	10
Football	90	10
Golf	95	5
Gymnastics	90	10
Ice skating	80	20
Racquetball	80	20
Rowing	20	80
Skiing	80	20
Squash	80	20
Soccer	60	40
Tennis	70	30
Volleyball	90	10

Table 29   To use interval training for a specific sport, you should select your work intervals according to the proportions suggested in this table.

along the lines of the first two weeks of our running programs in Chapter Four. (See Table 30.) You could do the
running program at the same time as your weight training
or calisthenics. It makes little difference whether you do
one before the other.

3. You should also take part in some sports and games purely
for relaxation and enjoyment. For example, a baseball
player might enjoy, and derive a conditioning benefit
from, squash or racquetball during the winter months.

4. If you have access to the proper facilities, you might also
practice a few of the skills needed for your sport. For
example, basketballers might do a little shooting, drib-
bling, pivoting and so on.

An Off-season Running I.T. Program

Week	Runs	Distance (yards)
1	4	220
	8	110
2	2	440
	8	110
3	2	440
	6	220
4	1	880
	6	220
5	2	880
	2	440
6	6	440
7	3	880
8	1	1½ miles

Table 30   Each workout should be done no more than twice a week at an
easy pace, with relief intervals that are three times as long as the time for each
run.

Preseason Training Using I.T.

In the eight to ten weeks before the season starts, the athlete should be preparing by using a specific eight-week (three workouts per week), high-intensity I.T. program. You can use any of the programs listed in the preceding few chapters, but most likely, running will be the best form of training for most sports. However, the running programs of Chapter Four are designed for general conditioning and have most of their emphasis on the development of the aerobic energy systems. If you intend to participate in a sport whose demands are mainly anaerobic, we suggest you modify those programs by substituting shorter-distance runs that will improve the capacity of your anaerobic systems.

The kind of adjustments that should be made in the sample programs given in the earlier chapters will obviously depend on the individual athlete, the sport or even the position within that sport, the initial fitness level of the athlete, and the types of movement needed during performance of the sport. Here are a few suggestions: besides adjusting the work rate, your coach might want to add to the total distance run or swum in each workout; football players might want to add some movement patterns common in football, such as the lateral and backward running that is characteristic of halfbacks and fullbacks; the substitutes for the work interval, again depending on the specific sport involved, might include such activities as skipping, hopping, rope jumping while running, skipping or hopping upstairs and wind sprints.

We would definitely not recommend that the training frequency, in these high-intensity programs, be increased from three to five days per week, no matter what the sport. Our research has shown us that in terms of increasing energy capacity, an interval training frequency of only two or three days per week is just as effective as five days per week and, not unnaturally, exhaustion is the enemy of training. If your coach wants you to attend training sessions five or six days a week, then the other two or three days should consist of much less intensive work. For example, you might watch game films or work on skills and strategies that are less strenuous than those you use during your I.T. workouts.

In this book, we can't give you preseason I.T. program examples for every sport and every sports activity. However, Table 29 shows you the percentages of anaerobic and aerobic activity that are desirable in I.T. programs for a variety of sports. You can use this table and the guidelines in the earlier chapters for running, swimming, weight training and so on. You will notice a couple of important omissions from the table: swimming and diving, which we mentioned in Chapter Five, and track and field, which we covered in Chapter Four.

It is especially important that the athlete warm up properly for an I.T. workout. We suggest you use the warm-up exer-

26. Arm sprints

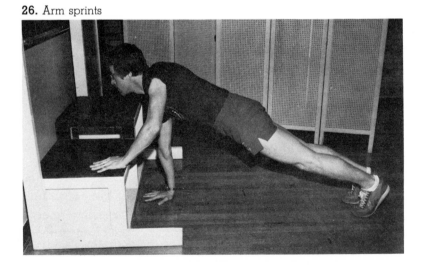

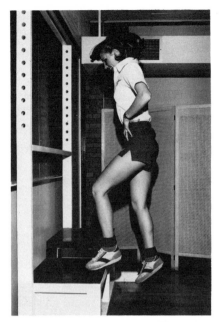

27. Bench blasts
grip power

cises of Chapter Three. However, though push-ups and sit-ups
are excellent warm-up exercises for athletes as well as nonathletes, you might want to use other exercises, which are
attuned to your sport. For example, most sports require more
arm and shoulder girdle power, leg power, and grip power
than is necessary for general conditioning. Depending on
your sport, you might want to modify the warm-up program by
using arm sprints, bench blasts or a grip exercise.

In-Season Training with I.T.

Traditionally, in-season training for most sports consists of
skills development. Most coaches feel that drills, practice
sessions and competition will maintain the level of fitness
obtained during preseason training. For the athletes who
work out seriously three times a week, we agree that drills,
practice sessions and competition will maintain a high level

of fitness throughout the season. However, we think that the skill drills for your sport should be done intervally so they will both improve your skills and build your energy capacity for that skill.

Let's take an example. Many sports use the "shuffle" drill, where the players move or shuffle as quickly as possible, first in one direction (left, right, front or back), then in another, continuously on command from the coach. Usually, this drill can be done only for a few minutes before exhaustion sets in. However, we think much more work could be done if the drill were performed intervally. Since the shuffle drill emphasizes power, the work interval should be between ten and thirty seconds. A suitable prescription might be five repetitions of the drill done in thirty seconds (for each drill), with a relief interval of one and a half minutes. Such a drill would take only ten minutes, would do more work than is usually achieved with the continuous form and yet would result in less overall fatigue.

Naturally, there are similar skill drills for all popular sports. In the next few pages, we'll take a look at the energy demands of a variety of sports and the skill drills that could be used for interval training in those sports.

Badminton

The game of badminton—the serious indoor variety, not the beach and backyard version—is a succession of sudden starts and stops that places great demands on the anaerobic capacity of your muscles. Unlike tennis, however, the action is quite continuous, so badminton also requires quite considerable stamina. Thus badminton players should use an off-season interval training program that includes running at both long and short distances.

Since badminton also calls for considerable flexibility in the shoulder, arm, and wrist, exercises to develop those muscles are an important part of a training program. Such exercises as push-ups, arm sprints and grip squeezes can help.

Most badminton players will be able to devise skill drills that can be done intervally to help in-season training. Here is one suggestion: With your practice partner, hit a high lob or overhead clear from deep in the other court, run quickly up to the net, touch it with your racquet and then run back to take your practice partner's return lob. This exercise will develop anaerobic capacity if done intervally for between ten and thirty seconds, with a relief interval three times as long as the time for one work interval.

Baseball

What energy systems are most needed by the baseball player? If we think about base running, hitting, throwing, pitching, catching, and fielding, it's clear that baseball's highest energy demands occur in a time of less than ten to twenty seconds. So I.T. prescriptions for baseball players should be mostly anaerobic.

The sport calls for arm, shoulder and leg muscle power for distance hitting, throwing and base running. So a baseball player should have a training program that includes bench stepping, arm sprints, push-ups and chin-ups, all done intervally. Pitchers, in particular, should do bench blasts to develop leg power for throwing.

There are many baseball drills that can be done intervally. For example, the baseball scramble develops skill in fielding ground balls and conditions anaerobically. In the baseball scramble drill, the coach, using a large supply of balls, hits or throws ground balls to a player, requiring him to move to his right and left continuously. Upon fielding the ball, the player throws to the coach's assistant.

Basketball

Abrupt starts and stops, jumping and short sprints require a basketball player to be well endowed with anaerobic power. At the same time, the lengthy periods of play, with little relief, produce fatigue through demands on the lactic acid system. Consequently, some aerobic conditioning should be part of the basketball player's I.T. program. However, we know that short-duration, high-intensity workouts do also develop the aerobic systems. Thus, most of a basketball player's I.T. program should be made up of anaerobic workouts.

Arm and shoulder power can be developed through an I.T. program using weight training, arm sprints, speed push-ups or

27A. An I.T. program for basketball players can increase anaerobic capacity for sprints and jumps while boosting arm and leg muscle power at the same time.

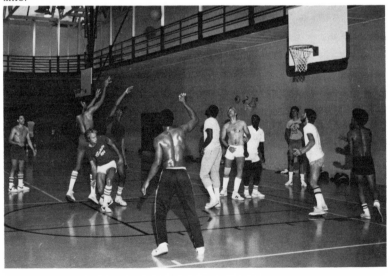

speed chin-ups. Leg power in basketball is also important, so your program might also include bench blasts, hopping up stairs, rope jumping and so on.

A good, vigorous skill drill in basketball is an exercise in which one player attempts to guard another. The offensive player (without a ball) tries to outmaneuver the defensive player. This is sometimes called the "mirror-image" drill. The work intervals should consist of all-out maneuvering for twenty to thirty seconds.

Another excellent I.T. skill drill, this time involving rebounding and tip-in skills, is as follows: To start, one player throws the ball against the backboard. As the ball rebounds, the other player jumps and taps the ball against the backboard, continuing to do so for ten to twenty seconds. If the second player loses control of the ball, the first player immediately puts another ball into play.

Cross-Country Skiing

The sport of cross-country skiing is one of the most rigorous endurance events. Successful cross-country skiers have some of the highest aerobic capacities ever measured (more than six liters of oxygen per minute, compared with three and a half for a normally healthy nonathlete of the same age). There's no question that the cross-country skier should follow a running I.T. program, with most of the emphasis on the longer distances to develop aerobic power.

For leg strength, the cross-country skier should use an I.T. program with bench blasts and flexibility exercises. A full warm-up program is also essential. In the low temperatures to be found during cross-country skiing, it is important to be thoroughly warmed up before competing or practicing.

Fencing

Fencing is another fast-moving sport that calls mostly for anaerobic power, though lengthy competitive fencing, particularly in such events as the saber, puts considerable demands on the aerobic system too.

I.T. programs for fencing should stress development of the legs, arms, and shoulders through speed push-ups, chin-ups, wrist curls and arm sprints. Bench blasts, running stadium steps, squat thrusts and leg presses can be used for strengthening and increasing the power of the leg muscles. However, an I.T. program for fencing might also be structured around running short distances in the work intervals. Rope jumping and running would be a fine combination for the fencing athlete. Stretching exercises are also important for the fencer and should be practiced before each workout. Good examples would include lunge stretches, lunge and arm stretches, and toe touching.

The lunge is an excellent example of a drill that will develop both a specific skill and anaerobic power. As a two-count exercise, an I.T. prescription for lunging might have ten repetitions of twenty lunges, with each repetition to be done in ten seconds and a thirty-second relief interval between repetitions. The lunges should be done as rapidly as possible. You should have your weapon in hand and a target to aim for. You can also do advance-retreat drills by working in fours. One fencer performs with weapon in hand while the others take their relief intervals. One of the resting fencers could call commands to the practicing fencer.

Football

If you were to pick a sport in which power was essential, football would be high, if not first, on the list. For example, several outstanding professional backs have had measured power outputs of between three and three and a half horsepower (with an average body weight of over 200 pounds). By contrast, the average man of the same age has a power output of about two horsepower. There's no wonder that professional scouts rely on the time for the 40-yard dash when selecting prospective candidates. The average time for the 40-yard dash for the same group of backs was 4.59 seconds. The back with the fastest time (4.35 seconds) also had the most power (3.5 horsepower).

Quite obviously, a training program for footballers must emphasize anaerobic power development. Besides preseason I.T. sprints, the program should have a selection of such exercises as bench blasts, arm sprints, speed push-ups, sit-ups and chin-ups, running stadium steps, and squat thrusts. Before the I.T. workout, a few flexibility exercises involving neck, shoulders, back, hips, and ankles should be practiced. Several years ago, we put a professional football player on a three-day-per-week sprint I.T. program eight weeks prior to his reporting to camp. He asserted: "I've never been in better shape for playing, either in college or professionally."

Interval weight training can be useful for football players mainly during the off-season, but could continue into the preseason for those who are unfit. The weight training exercises should concentrate on arm, shoulder and leg power.

There are many skill drills in football that lend themselves to interval training. For example, most of the blocking drills against the sled can be done intervally. A good starting prescription might be all-out hitting and driving for ten repetitions of five seconds of effort, with fifteen seconds of relief.

Golf
Very few golf books or magazines discuss or even mention

training programs for golf fitness. Yet development of power in both arms can give you greater distances on the fairways. Sprints, bench blasts, chin-ups or push-ups done intervally will give you a more powerful golf stroke. A sprint program would be satisfactory for general conditioning. With such a program you should also include such exercises as chin-ups, speed push-ups, arm sprints or weight training exercises to develop arms and shoulders.

Grip power is another important factor in controlling the club, so interval tennis ball squeezing should be a part of your program too. You might also incorporate stretching exercises in your warm-up program to promote flexibility of the trunk, shoulders, arms and neck.

Gymnastics

Competitive gymnastics requires great muscular flexibility, strength and power. It is a sport that lends itself to the methods of interval training and one in which the participants can gain much by using I.T. Obviously, a great deal of time should be spent with interval weight training, although some sprinting, particularly for those involved with floor exercises, is also recommended. Special weight training devices can be built so the exercises can be performed with controlled overloading and through the same movements found in gymnastic routines.

Gymnastics is an ideal sport for I.T. skill drills. Most gymnastic routines can be isolated and repeated to an interval schedule. For example, a drill might consist of performing repeated muscle-ups to press handstands. This could be done intervally with, say, ten repetitions of as many muscle-ups as can be done in ten seconds, each repetition to be followed by a thirty-second relief interval. An Olympic hopeful should probably perform sixty full routines per day. Some Japanese

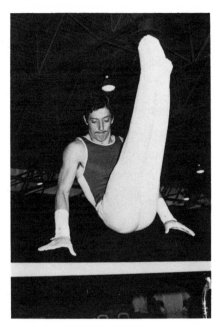

27B. Most gymnastic routines can be done to an I.T. schedule so skills and physical fitness can be improved with the same effort.

gymnasts do as many as two hundred per day. The choice is up to you, but you will get more from your workouts if you do the exercises intervally.

Ice Hockey

Ice hockey is one of the fastest sports played by man. The forwards and defense men need to develop both anaerobic and aerobic systems since they will not only have to skate very rapidly at times but will skate some three miles in the course of a game. About 80 percent of the three miles involves quick breaks at very high speeds, particularly for the forwards. These quick breaks are often done more than fifty times in a game.

Even though hockey does not involve running, we feel that an I.T. program based on sprint running could be useful.

However, a similar program on the ice would be equally beneficial. So you could design an I.T. program of short sprints on the ice, both forward and backward.

The arm, shoulder, wrist, and grip are important in hockey because of stick control and body checks. So we'd also recommend a program that includes strength and power I.T. prescriptions using one or more of weights, calisthenics, bench blasts, arm sprints, and ball squeezing.

Skill drills that could be incorporated into an I.T. program could include a variation of the mirror-image drill suggested for basketball players or relay drills with and without the puck. These are all excellent drills for combining improvement in skills and fitness.

Racquetball

In the last few years, racquetball has grown by leaps and bounds, a statement that also characterizes the sport. Played in a walled court similar to a squash court, racquetball calls for power in the arms, shoulders, and wrist to hit the ball and power in the legs to run quickly around the court. Thus the sport places great demands on the anaerobic systems. Unlike, say, tennis, the game can be practiced individually, with the player hitting against himself by taking every ball as it rebounds. Racquetball is ideally suited to I.T. programs for both general conditioning and skill drills.

A racquetball I.T. program should be based on running, with the emphasis on sprints. Part of the program could be short forward and back and lateral runs within the court itself. The program should contain a few longer runs to build up the aerobic systems, which would come into play in a long match.

Muscular strength and flexibility are important for the racquetballer, who should use the warm-up exercises of Chapter

Three, with bench blasts and arm sprints to strengthen the arm and leg muscles. Grip exercises using an old or a dead racquetball ball will help add extra gripping power. Although the racquet used in the sport is quite light, the forces involved in hitting the ball are severe. The forehand drive or "kill" of professional champion Marty Hogan has been measured at over 130 miles per hour.

I.T. skill drills in racquetball can easily be designed to suit a particular player. For example, you could hit a lob or "ceiling" ball down the side wall of the court, run over to the opposite side wall and back to hit another ceiling ball as the ball returns to the back wall. A typical I.T. prescription might be ten repetitions of five ceiling balls done in ten seconds, with a thirty-second relief interval between repetitions.

Rowing

The rower has perhaps the most demanding physical job of any athlete. Both arms and legs must be pushed to the limits for periods of up to six minutes (eight-oared shell, 2000-meter event for men). Thus rowing requires development of both aerobic and anaerobic energy systems.

The question arises as to whether training programs for rowers should be land- or water-based. We feel that power is probably developed more by rowing and specific weight training exercises (those simulating stroke movements) than by running. On the other hand, running is perhaps the best way of developing your aerobic capacity. So I.T. programs for oarsmen and women should consist of weight training, rowing, and running. Bench blasts might also be useful for leg muscle strength.

Rowing calls for skills in timing and the application of power that can easily be adapted to interval routines. It should be an easy matter to develop rowing skill drills that can be performed intervally.

Skiing

Slalom, jumping, downhill and pleasure skiing depend mainly on the anaerobic energy systems, unlike cross-country skiing, which is largely an aerobic sport. An I.T. program for skiers should consist of sprint running and bench blasts to strengthen the leg muscles. A downhill skier should also do flexibility exercises for the ankles and hips. Ankle movements that point the toes, bend the foot and rotate it should be practiced.

Squash

Like racquetball, squash is a game of quick starts and sudden stops. Rather more power is needed to hit a squash ball, which is harder than the racquetball ball. Thus squash is mostly an anaerobic sport, although aerobic endurance does play a significant part, particularly in the longer singles matches.

A squash I.T. program should probably be based on running prescriptions, with the emphasis on the shorter distances. However, the program should also contain some longer runs to build up the aerobic systems, which would be used in longer matches. The I.T. program might also have some weight training exercises to build muscular strength in the shoulders, arms and wrist. Bench blasts might be useful to build up the leg muscles too.

Since squash is played in a walled court, the strokes of the game can be practiced alone. Such practice routines can also be done intervally and incorporated into a squash player's I.T. program. For example, you could hit angled drives from deep in the court from forehand to backhand side, so you would have to run across the court to return each shot; or you could hit alternate hard and soft shots to force yourself to run the length of the court between hits. Any squash player will, no doubt, have favorite routines that can be done intervally.

Soccer

Soccer is an example of a sport where the position played affects the energy needs of each player. For example, full-back and goalkeeper are strictly power positions, so an I.T. program for such players would be based on the anaerobic systems. By contrast, the forwards work about half the field and so should develop both the aerobic and anaerobic sys-

27C. Soccer players need both aerobic and anaerobic capacity which are best developed by an I.T. program that combines skill drills with an endurance activity such as running.

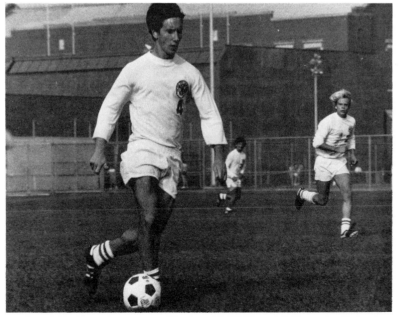

tems. In terms of aerobic endurance, the toughest position is that of the halfback, who spends much of the game running the length of the field. Halfbacks need to develop their aerobic energy systems.

There are many skill drills in soccer that can be adapted to interval training. A good example is the so-called pressure drill. In this drill, a player dribbles back and forth over a distance of 30 to 40 yards, keeping the ball under control for ten to thirty seconds. Another drill that involves kicking accuracy is the "scramble" drill, in which the coach, well supplied with balls, kicks them to right, left, and center at random, causing the player to move rapidly across the field while kicking the balls at a predetermined target. The work interval for this routine should be twenty to thirty seconds.

Tennis

Training for tennis, as most coaches will agree, is highly individualistic, requiring considerable personal motivation. Tennis is essentially an anaerobic sport, so an I.T. program should include intervals of short, high-intensity work. Harry Hopman, the coach of many successful Australian Davis Cup teams, was a firm believer in the value of conditioning for tennis players. Hopman's program for his players consisted of many short wind sprints followed by groups of calisthenics, particularly exercises to speed up footwork and strengthen the leg muscles. Such a program could, and should, be done intervally.

Dr. John Hendrix, former Ohio State University tennis coach and former director of the National Junior Davis Cup training camp, favors the use of 40-yard sprints for young tennis players. Development of arm, shoulder, grip, and leg power via weight training, arm sprints, bench blasts, and similar I.T. exercises will also improve tennis performance.

For a tennis skill drill that can be done intervally, Dr. Hendrix recommends the tennis scramble, in which the coach feeds balls from the net position to a player on the baseline. Balls are fed left, right and center at random, with the player returning to the center position after each shot. The coach can also hit balls short to force the player to come up to the net and then retreat again. The player, of course, should be hitting to a target. This drill can be done with several players by having a player on either side of the coach volleying back the baseliner's shots. Since those players move very little, they can be taking their relief intervals in those positions.

Volleyball

Power volleyball is another example of an almost purely anaerobic sporting activity. As in basketball, leg power (for vertical jumping) is a vital attribute that the coach should try to develop. A running I.T. program should be useful for the volleyballer, provided that it consists mainly of sprinting. Similarly, weight training should consist of short, rapid, high-intensity lifts done to an interval schedule. Such lifts might consist of knee bends and toe raises. Other leg power exercises might include a rapid succession of vertical jumps and bench blasts.

There are many excellent skill drills in volleyball that can be done intervally. The drills should emphasize movement, both lateral and forward and back. A three-on-one drill with three players on one side of the net throwing to one player on the other side will provide plenty of exercise in short intervals. The players can rotate and take their relief intervals by throwing to the single defending player. Such an exercise should be done in intervals of twenty to thirty seconds.

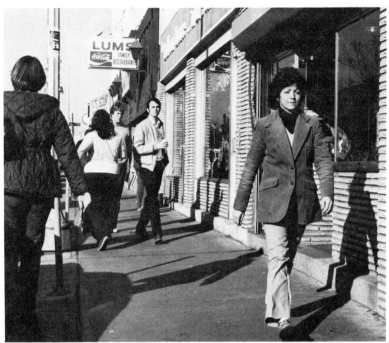

28. Although you can become fit quickly through interval training, you should also make your life-style active, for example, by walking wherever possible.

9 HOW TO TAKE CARE OF YOUR BODY

Change Your Life-style to Keep Fit

Keeping fit is not merely a matter of exercising several times a week: you should orient your life to treating your body properly and helping yourself stay in shape. There are two simple principles to follow: first, take every opportunity you can to exercise your body outside your regular interval training program; and second, give your body the best chance of performing well by eating, drinking, and sleeping properly. You need not be a fanatic to follow these two principles. Only a few changes will be needed for most of you.

As your level of fitness improves, you'll probably find that you become more active in your everyday life. Mowing the lawn, painting the house or vacuum cleaning won't seem quite the tiring chores they used to be. But remember you can apply the principles of interval training to household tasks too. Mow strenuously for a few minutes and then rest or do some less arduous activity like pruning for a few minutes. You'll find the lawn mowing or housecleaning goes much more easily the interval way.

You should also look out for other simple ways of using your body. When you drop the car off at the shop for repairs, why not walk to your next destination? Allow yourself a little extra time, walk briskly, and you'll feel better for it (both physically and spiritually, no doubt). When you need that extra half gallon of milk, why not bike down to the store? Stuck in a traffic jam? Carry an old tennis ball in your car so you can squeeze it to strengthen your wrist and arm muscles. When the kids are playing Frisbee in the yard, don't switch on the television; go out and play. You'll enjoy it just as much as the children. And you'll be doing yourself some good into the bargain. Eventually, a more active life-style will seem quite natural to you.

Eating for Personal Fitness

The amount of food you need for personal fitness will depend on how active you are. Just as an auto that travels 100 miles in a day needs more gas than one that travels 10 miles, so a person walking 20 miles per day needs more food than one walking two miles. Everyone needs a certain amount of food for body maintenance and growth, but over that amount, your food intake should be approximately equal to your energy needs. If you eat more than you need, you'll put on weight. If you eat less, you'll lose weight over a period of time.

With most Americans, the problem is not eating too little. The difficulty is that many of us eat too much of the wrong types of food. Convenience foods may satisfy a craving to eat, but they often do not provide enough of the energy needs of the physically active individual. We are not going to give you a specific diet, nor do we believe in prescribing diets for weight loss (or gain). Just as we suggested you should formulate your own exercise program, we feel you should be able to devise your own diet to meet your needs (which, of course, are different from those of other individuals).

The essential energy nutrients are proteins, fats, and carbohydrates. The primary nutrients that provide muscular energy are fats and carbohydrates. Protein is not usually an energy nutrient, but it will promote cell and tissue growth and repair in the body. A balanced diet for a normally active individual should have about 10–15 percent protein, 25–30

Natural Foods*

Fat	Carbohydrate	Protein
Bacon	Baked Beans	Cereal
Butter	Bread	Cheese
Margarine	Cakes	Eggs
Nuts	Cereals	Fish
Peanut Butter	Dried Fruits	Lean Meat
Pork	Fresh Fruits	Milk
Salad Oils	Honey	Nuts
	Pastries	Poultry
	Potatoes	Soy Beans
	Syrup	Vegetables
	Vegetables	(legumes)

Table 31
*From E. L. Fox, *Sports Physiology* (Philadelphia: W. B. Saunders, 1979).

percent fat and 55–60 percent carbohydrate. Table 31 gives you some examples of natural foods in each of the three essential categories.

Good eating habits entail knowing how to select foods and how many meals to eat per day. For a properly balanced diet, you should select specific foods from each of the following four food groups: milk and milk products; meat and high-protein foods; fruits and vegetables; cereal and grain foods. The American Association for Health, Physical Education and Recreation has broken down the essential food groups even further into milk, meat (including fish, poultry, cheese, and eggs), dark green or deep yellow vegetables, citrus fruits, other fruits and vegetables, bread (including cereals and potatoes), fats and sugars. Table 32 lists food groups from which you may select your daily diet. You will see that the range of foods is very wide, although the quantities may be smaller than those you might normally consume. You do not need special meals to eat properly—just the right amounts of the proper food groups (see the daily food guide, Table 33).

Foods Which Within a Group May Be Exchanged for Each Other*

Food Groups

Milk

(1 cup whole milk contains 12 grams carbohydrate, 8 grams protein, 10 grams fat, and 170 calories; 1 cup of skim milk contains 80 calories; 1 cup cocoa made with milk contains approx. 200 calories.)

1 cup whole milk
1 cup skim milk
½ cup evaporated milk
¼ cup powdered milk
1 cup buttermilk
1 cup cocoa

Meat Group

(1 ounce contains 7 grams protein, 5 grams fat, and 75 calories.)

1 ounce lean beef, lamb, pork, liver, chicken*
1 ounce fish—cod, haddock, perch, etc.
1 hot dog
¼ cup tuna, salmon, crab, lobster
5 small oysters, shrimp, clams
3 medium sardines
1 slice cheese
¼ cup cottage cheese
1 egg
2 tablespoons peanut butter

*1 average serving of meat or fish (such as a pork chop or 2 meatballs) is about 3 ounces.

Dark Green or Deep Yellow Vegetables (½ cup is one serving)

(Greens and lettuce have very little carbohydrate content. The other vegetables contain approximately 7 grams carbohydrate and 2 grams protein and 35 calories.)

Broccoli*	Greens*
Carrots	Beet greens
Chicory*	Chard
Escarole*	Collard
Pepper	Kale
Pumpkin	Mustard
Tomatoes*	Spinach
Watercress*	Turnip greens
Winter squash	Lettuce*

*Low-calorie vegetables.

Citrus Fruits or Substitute (½ cup is one serving)

(The carbohydrate is averaged to approximately 10 grams per ½ cup and 40 calories.)

Orange	Grapefruit juice*	Tangerine
Orange juice	Cantaloupe*	Tomato juice*
Grapefruit*		

*Low-calorie fruits.

Other Fruits and Vegetables

Fruits (½ cup is approx. 10 grams carbohydrate and 40 calories.)

Apple	Dates	Pear
Applesauce	Figs	Pineapple
Apricots	Grapes	Plums
Banana (½ small)	Grape juice (¼ cup)	Raisins (2 tablespoons)
Raspberries	Honeydew melon	Pineapple juice (⅓ cup)
Blueberries	Mango	Prunes (2 medium)
Cherries	Papaya	Watermelon*
	Peach	

*Low-calorie fruits.

Vegetables (½ cup is one serving.)

(The vegetables without the asterisk contain approximately 7 grams carbohydrate, 2 grams protein, and 35 calories.)

Asparagus*	Cucumbers*	Radishes*
Beets	Eggplant*	Rutabagas
Brussels sprouts*	Mushrooms*	Sauerkraut*
Cabbage*	Okra*	String beans*
Cauliflower*	Onions	Summer squash*
Celery*	Peas, green	Turnips

*Low-calorie fruits and vegetables

Bread Group

(1 slice of bread or 1 substitute contains 15 grams carbohydrate, 2 grams protein, and 70 calories.)

½ hamburger bun
½ hot dog bun
1 cup popcorn
2½" wedge pizza
1 slice enriched
   bread
1 biscuit or roll
1 small muffin
1 small piece
   cornbread
½ cup cooked
   cereal
¾ cup ready-to-eat
   cereal

½ cup spaghetti,
   noodles, macaroni,
   etc.
2 graham crackers
5 saltines
6 round, thin
   crackers
½ cup beans or
   peas (dried or
   cooked)
   (lima or navy
   beans, split pea,
   cowpeas, etc.)
¼ cup baked beans
⅓ cup corn
½ cup rice or grits

⅔ cup parsnips
1 small potato
½ cup mashed
   potato
15 potato chips—1
   ounce bag
6 pretzels, medium,
   or 20 thin sticks
8 French fries
½ cup sweet
   potatoes or yams
1½" cube sponge
   or angel cake (no
   icing)
½ cup ice cream
   (omit 2 fat
   servings)

Fat Group

(1 teaspoon fat contains 5 grams fat and 45 calories.)

Bacon (1 slice)   Cream cheese (1 tbsp.)

Butter or margarine (1 tsp.)   French dressing (1 tbsp.)
Cream, light (2 tbsp.)   Mayonnaise (1 tsp.)
Cream, heavy—40% (1 tbsp.)   Oil or cooking fat (1 tsp.)

Sugars

(1 teaspoon contains 5 grams carbohydrate and 20 calories.)

Sugar   Syrup
Jelly   Hard candy
Honey   Carbonated beverage (¼ cup)
Note: Salt used in the home should be iodized.

Table 32
   *From *Nutrition for the Athlete* (Washington, D.C.: American Association
for Health, Physical Education and Recreation).

Daily Food Guide*

Food Group	Daily Amounts	Main Contribution
I. Milk and cheese	Teen-agers: 4 or more cups Adults: 2 or more cups	Calcium Protein Riboflavin Vitamin D
II. Meat: Beef, veal, pork, lamb, poultry, fish, eggs	2 or more servings Serving size: 2–3 ounces lean, boneless	Protein Thiamin Iron
Alternates: Dry beans, dry peas, lentils, nuts, peanut butter	cooked meat, poultry, fish 2 eggs	
	1 cup cooked dry beans, dry peas or lentils 4 tablespoons peanut butter	Niacin Riboflavin
III. Bread and cereals (whole-grain or enriched)	4 or more servings Serving size: 1 slice bread	Thiamin Riboflavin Niacin

	½–¾ cup cooked cereal, macaroni, or spaghetti 1 ounce (1 cup) ready-to-eat cereal 5 saltines or 2 graham crackers	Iron Protein
IV. Vegetables and fruits	4 or more servings Serving size: ½ cup dark green or deep yellow every other day	Vitamin A
	½ cup or 1 medium citrus fruit (or any raw fruit or vegetable rich in ascorbic acid)	Ascorbic acid
	Other vegetables and fruit including potato (1 medium)	Other vitamins and minerals
Water	6 to 8 glasses	

Table 33

*From M. Krause, and M. Hunscher, *Food, Nutrition and Diet Therapy,* 5th ed. (Philadelphia: W. B. Saunders, 1972).

It's also very important to eat regularly. If you are to follow an active life-style, your energy level must be kept up. As you consume energy by exercising, your blood glucose levels will drop. When they drop too low, you will feel tired and there will be some loss of efficiency. Depending on the amount of activity that you do, you'll begin to experience some fatigue within three hours of eating, so it's important to get at least three proper meals a day. It's especially important to begin your day with a proper breakfast even if you sit at a desk all day. An example of a basic three-meal diet is given in Table 34. You can supplement this diet with snacks to make a five-meal diet, provided that the snacks contribute to your proper nutrition (see Table 34).

Basic Diets in Three and Five Meals*

5 Meals	3 Meals
Breakfast	**Breakfast**
½ grapefruit ⅔ cup bran flakes 1 cup skim or low-fat milk or other beverage	½ cup orange juice 1 soft-boiled or poached egg 1 slice whole wheat toast 1½ teaspoons margarine 1 cup skim or low-fat milk or other beverage
Snack	
1 small package raisins ½ bologna sandwich	
Lunch	**Lunch**
1 slice pizza 1 serving of carrot sticks 1 apple 1 cup skim or low-fat milk	1½ cup Manhattan clam chowder 2 rye wafers ½ cup cottage cheese (uncreamed) 1 medium bunch grapes or 1 medium apple 1 granola cookie
Snack	
2 oatmeal cookies	

Dinner

1 baked fish with
       mushroom (3 ounces)
1 baked potato
2 teaspoons margarine
½ cup broccoli
1 cup tomato juice or skim
       or low-fat milk

Dinner

1 helping of oven-
       barbecued chicken
       (3 ounces, no bone)
½ cup green beans
½ cup cabbage and
       carrot salad
⅔ cup mashed potato
½ cup applesauce
1 cup skim or low-fat
       milk or other
       beverage

Total calories: about 1400   Total calories: about 1200

Table 34   *From N. J. Smith, *Food for Sport* (Palo Alto, Calif.: Bull Publishing, 1976).

You'll see that the typical diets we've listed contain about 1200–1400 calories, which is sufficient for the normal adult but not for the growing child or the active athlete. We'll have more to say about eating for athletes later in this chapter. These diets are adequate for an adult who exercises regularly but does not have a physically active occupation. If your job is an active one, you'll need more calories from the food groups we've recommended.

Weight Loss and Exercise
Obesity is a major problem among both adults and children in the U.S. today. It's commonly supposed that exercise will lead to weight loss. While this is certainly true, few people understand that a tremendous amount of exercise is needed

to lose even one pound. For example, about six hours of cross-country running at a fairly stiff pace might lose a pound of fat from a normal adult. You can lose weight much more easily by restricting your food intake and exercising regularly. However, obesity is best controlled by prevention, particularly at an early age. Proper diet in preadolescence will do much to prevent obesity in later years.

The amount of body fat stored in a person is determined by the number of fat-storing cells and the capacity of those cells. The number of fat cells cannot be reduced by exercise or dietary restrictions once adulthood is reached. However, exercise and diet programs introduced in early childhood can lead to a reduction in both the number and the size of the fat cells during the adult years. So it's important that your children eat properly and exercise regularly to develop living habits that will stay with them for a lifetime. Though an overweight adult cannot reduce the number of fat cells in his or her body, he or she can reduce their size by restricting food (caloric) intake.

How much should you weigh? Table 35 presents suggested ranges of weights by height and age for men and women. Most experts feel that the normal body weight between the ages of twenty-five and thirty should not be exceeded throughout life. If you wish to lose weight, we suggest that you do so by reducing your food intake and exercising regularly. On a diet of 1000 to 1200 calories per day, most adults will lose about one or two pounds a week, provided they exercise. Just as an exercise program takes several weeks to bring an inactive body back into shape, a controlled diet can take many weeks to bring body weight into line. There are no shortcuts to weight loss, despite the number of popular books on the subject. Looking after your body is a major lifetime commitment.

Best Weight (pounds, in indoor clothing)

| | | Men | |
Height	Age 20–24	Age 25–29	Age 30–39
5'2"	124	127	129
5'5"	133	136	140
5'8"	147	150	153
5'11"	158	163	166
6'2"	174	177	181

| | | Women | |
Height	Age 20–24	Age 25–29	Age 30–39
4'11"	104	107	109
5'2"	114	116	118
5'5"	122	124	127
5'8"	134	135	138
5'10"	142	143	148

Table 35   Many insurance companies develop "best weight" tables. It's the weight they believe Americans *should weigh*, not the actual average weights of Americans. This is the "best weight" table developed by the Pacific Mutual Life Insurance Co. The weights in the table are 10 percent less than actual average weights.

Diet and the Athlete

The foods an athlete eats are important because an ordinary diet can impose definite limits on performance. Simply stated, if an athlete does not eat enough, he will grow tired faster and so perform badly. But too much food can result in too much fat. There are other considerations for the athlete. For example, the foods eaten before and after an event can be chosen to help the athlete's performance. And the diet can be manipulated to load the glycogen stores in the muscles.

	Age 40–49	Age 50–59	Age 60–69
	130	131	130
	142	143	142
	155	156	155
	167	168	167
	183	184	181

	Age 40–49	Age 50–59	Age 60–69
	114	117	120
	122	127	129
	132	137	139
	142	146	147
	151	154	155

The amount of food needed by an athlete will vary considerably from person to person and from sport to sport. We can give only a few examples here. A young male athlete may be expending as much as 5000 calories per day in exercise which would call for a diet of around 6000 calories (see Table 36), taken in perhaps as many as six meals per day. Note the quality of food in this diet—low amounts of large-bulk foods (such as cereals, beverages and salads), low amounts of animal fats and an abundance of low-bulk car-

A High-calorie (6000 calories) Diet in Six Meals*

Breakfast

- ½ cup orange juice
- 1 cup oatmeal
- 1 cup low-fat milk
- 1 scrambled egg
- 1 slice whole wheat toast
- 1½ teaspoons margarine
- 1 tablespoon jam

Snack

- 1 peanut butter sandwich
- 1 banana
- 1 cup grape juice

Lunch

- 5 fish sticks with tartar sauce
- 1 large serving French fries
- 1 bowl of green salad with avocado and French dressing
- 1 cup lemon sherbet
- 2 granola cookies
- 1 cup low-fat milk

Snack

- 1 cup mixed dried fruit
- 1½ cup malted milk

Dinner

- 1 cup cream of mushroom soup
- 2 pieces oven-baked chicken
- 1 candied sweet potato
- 1 dinner roll and margarine
- 1 cup carrots and peas
- ½ cup cole slaw
- 1 piece cherry pie
- 1 beverage

Snack

- 1 cup cashew nuts
- 1 cup cocoa

Table 36

*From N. J. Smith, *Food for Sport* (Palo Alto, Calif.: Bull Publishing, 1976).

A Low-calorie (2000 calories) Diet in Five Meals*

Breakfast

½ cup orange juice
1 soft-boiled egg
1 slice whole wheat toast
2 teaspoons margarine
1 glass skim milk or other
    beverage

Snack

1 banana

Lunch

1 hamburger (3 ounces) on a
    roll with relish
½ sliced tomato
1 glass skim milk
1 medium apple

Snack

1 carton fruit-flavored
    yogurt
1 cup grape juice

Dinner

1 serving of baked chicken
    marengo (½ breast)
¾ cup rice
5-6 Brussels sprouts
1 bowl of green salad with
    French dressing
1 small piece gingerbread
1 cup skim milk or other
    beverage

Table 37
*From N. J. Smith, *Food for Sport* (Palo Alto, Calif. Bull Publishing, 1976).

bohydrates. At the other end of the scale, a young athlete who is overweight should adopt a low-calorie diet that will still permit daily physical exercise (see Table 37). A diet of around 2000 calories per day will produce a weight loss of about two or three pounds a week in an active athlete.

One of us (ELF) was studying the dietary habits of some of the Ohio State athletes several years ago. Part of the study involved asking them to recall, every few days, what and how much they had eaten. Most of the athletes ate about 5000 calories per day. However, one swimmer, in a single day, ate 15,000 calories' worth of food! That's about ten times what the normal young adult eats per day. By the way, the swimmer, over the period of the season, didn't gain a single pound.

For athletes in endurance sports such as long-distance running and cross-country skiing, performance can be significantly improved by increasing the stores of muscle glycogen. You can do this by following a high-carbohydrate diet for three or four days before the event, or by exercise-induced glycogen depletion followed by a three-day high-carbohydrate diet, or by exercise-induced glycogen depletion followed by a three-day diet high in fat and protein and then by a three-day high-carbohydrate diet. We don't have enough space to go into details here, but you'll find more information in *Sports Physiology* by Edward L. Fox (Philadelphia: W. B. Saunders, 1979).

Eating Before Performance
There are no "superfoods" that, taken before activity, will lead to "super" performances. Proper nutrition for both the athlete and the nonathlete is a year-round task. However, there are certain foods that should be avoided on the day of competition, such as meats that are digested slowly and may cause a feeling of fullness if eaten within four hours of the performance. You might also want to avoid gas-forming foods, greasy and highly seasoned foods.

Carbohydrates should be the major constituent of the pregame meal and should be consumed no later than two and a half hours before the competition. Carbohydrates are easily digested and help maintain the blood glucose levels. The pregame meal can also include moderate portions of such foods as fruits, cooked vegetables, gelatin desserts and fish.

Consumption of large amounts of glucose (sugar) in liquid or pill form less than an hour before exercise is not recommended. Too much sugar stimulates insulin production, so that blood-borne glucose is actually reduced during exercise. However, provided the sugar concentration is not excessive, liquids can be drunk up to thirty minutes before physical activity. Water is the best liquid, but fruit and vegetable juices are also suitable.

There are really no hard and fast rules about diet on the day of competition. Your diet should be the same as that normally consumed. However, you should remember that nervousness and tension during competition can affect the digestive system, so foods normally eaten without discomfort could cause some distress. Experience will tell you which foods to avoid. Provided you do not overeat or eat foods that cause stomach upsets, your performance will not be affected by using your normal diet for your pregame meal.

Water Loss During Exercise

During heavy physical activity, particularly on hot or humid days, large quantities of water and some salt are lost by the body through sweating. Heat illness may result if the water and salt are not replaced within twenty-four hours. The water loss is more serious than the salt (a normal diet will replace the salt without the need for salt tablets). Anyone who exercises on hot and humid days should be aware of the need to replenish the water lost.

An athlete may lose 5 to 15 pounds of water (one pint of water is equivalent to one pound) during physical activity over a period of one and a half to two hours. Unfortunately, the thirst mechanism—the natural desire for drinking water—is not always adequate to the task of replacing the fluid lost. So for an athlete, body weight measurements should be taken every day. Any significant weight loss after practicing or playing on a hot day could indicate the start of dehydration. Extra liquids, preferably cold water, should be taken. Another simple indicator of dehydration is the color of the urine. A light color would indicate that sufficient liquids are being consumed to replace those lost through sweating, while a dark color would indicate a need for water intake.

Heat Problems in Exercise

Although heat problems are more likely to occur in athletes who are asked to perform intensively under hot and humid conditions, nonathletes can suffer from excessive heat, particularly if they wear clothing that prevents evaporative cooling. The more body covering used, the less evaporative cooling will take place and the warmer the body will get with increasing activity. Heat stress will affect the cardiovascular system and increase the tendency to heat illness or even heat stroke. The latter can be fatal.

When exercising in hot and humid conditions, you should wear loose clothing that exposes much of the body to allow for sweating and, hence, cooling. You should not wear warm-up suits that are intended to cut off evaporative cooling. There is absolutely no place in exercise programs for rubberized suits. Such suits will raise body temperature and greatly increase the risk of heat illness.

You should also learn to recognize the symptoms of heat injury and the steps to take for immediate treatment. The usual warning symptoms are hair standing on end on chest and arms, chilling, throbbing pressure in the head, unsteadiness, nausea and dry skin. If heat exhaustion is allowed to become heat stroke, the sweating mechanism can fail and body temperature can rise to the point where irreversible changes occur. If you suspect heat illness in yourself or a colleague, immediate action is called for and you should arrange for emergency treatment by a physician or hospital.

The usual treatment for a victim of heat illness is to remove all the clothing and attempt cooling by whatever means available (such as a garden hose, containers of ice water or a cold shower). You should also immediately summon an emergency vehicle and notify the hospital of a possible heat casualty. En route to the hospital, use sponges or towels to apply ice water to the victim. With proper and prompt treatment, heat illness can be arrested and the victim revived.

Exercise and Muscular Injury

At one time or another, all of us have experienced muscle soreness. What causes muscular soreness is not exactly known, but we can suggest several ways to lessen the chances of soreness and to prevent the injury from becoming more serious. We think that soreness is most likely to be due to overstretching tendons. Muscle soreness seems to be most likely to occur when muscles are stretched—as, for example, in lifting a barbell. The tension developed during muscle extensions stretches the tissues associated with both the tendons and the muscle fibers.

You can deal with muscular soreness in two ways. First, by doing stretching exercises for the muscles concerned. Stretching appears to help not only in the prevention of soreness but also in the relief of sore muscles. Stretching exercises should be performed without bouncing or jerking, or more muscle damage may occur. Some suitable stretching exercises are given in Chapter Three, on warming up.

Second, some experts feel that taking vitamin C (ascorbic acid) for a period of about thirty days will prevent or at least reduce subsequent muscular soreness. The dose should be about 100 milligrams per day (twice the daily recommended normal dosage). The effectiveness of this treatment has not been entirely proved, although it seems to work for some athletes.

Of course, interval training significantly reduces the chance of muscular injury, because your muscles recover between work intervals. The risk of injury is highest when the body is tired from physically demanding work. With interval training, because the build-up of lactic acid in your bloodstream is lessened, you simply do not get as tired as you would with conventional continuous exercise. If you progress in your training program at the rates we recommend, it's very unlikely that you'll become excessively sore or damage a muscle by overexertion when you are tired.

First Aid and Emergencies

Anyone who exercises regularly runs some risk of injury. Fortunately, most exercise-related injuries are minor and require only first aid. The most common injuries are muscular soreness and sprains, cuts and bruises (as, for example, caused by slipping while running), and blisters (mostly from footwear that does not fit properly). Common sense and ordinary first aid can handle most of these problems.

Cuts and abrasions should be cleaned carefully with a mild antiseptic and then dressed with a sterile bandage. If bleeding is moderate, it can usually be stopped by elevating the limb concerned for a few minutes. However, if bleeding is severe or if you cannot clean the cut properly, you should seek the help of a physician immediately.

If you get a blister, do not break it. Clean and dry the foot and apply a "doughnut-shaped" dressing so the blister is surrounded. The dressing will help stop further friction on the blister. Hikers often use a leatherlike material called moleskin to surround a blister. You can obtain moleskin at a good pharmacy. If the blister breaks, carefully cut off the loose skin with sterile scissors, put a little antibiotic ointment on the wound and cover it with sterile gauze. You can then put a doughnut dressing over the sterile gauze.

Should you sprain a muscle or damage a joint, it's best to avoid using it and to seek medical advice right away. It's very tough to distinguish between an ankle sprain and a fracture without using X rays. Although a muscular sprain will often recover in a few days without specific treatment other than rest, it pays to be sure that you have nothing more serious than a sprain.

In the case of more serious injuries, do not go beyond simple first aid unless you have had specific paramedical training. In a true emergency, make the victim as comfortable and as warm as you can, and send for help immediately. Reassurance to the victim is often the most important help you can give until more qualified assistance arrives. Above all, try to remain calm and act methodically.

Of course, we hope that you will never be faced with serious injury in the course of exercising. As in most activities, accidents and injury can often be prevented by carrying out the activities in a sensible and planned manner. A little care and forethought will pay off in the prevention of injuries while exercising.

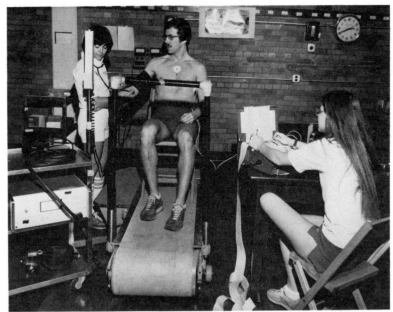

29. If you haven't exercised before, it's best to get a thorough physical exam before you start.

10 HOW TO CHECK YOURSELF OUT

Know Your Own Body

Just as you can tell when you have overeaten, so you will be able to gauge, in general terms, your physical fitness. Indeed, the feeling of well-being that comes from a proper physical training program is so strong that it will become your principal motivator for continuing with your exercises. And if you have to stop your training program because of injury or illness, the desire to achieve, once again, that feeling of fitness will be a powerful motivator in your recovery.

However, if you have never exercised before on a regular basis, there's every chance that you may overdo things in your enthusiasm to get in shape. So we suggest you get a full physical examination from your physician before you start an exercise program. You should do this no matter what your age if you have not previously led an active life. However, even if you think you are fit, we recommend that anyone over the age of thirty-five get a thorough physical—and clearance from a physician—before starting an I.T. program.

Once you enter into your training program, your body will begin to tell you how you are doing, but we feel that you may wish to have more precise methods of measuring your performance. There are many tests, ranging from simple pulse taking to complex cardiovascular tests, that you can do for yourself with nothing more than a stopwatch (and some patience). In this chapter, we'll show you some of the more useful tests and how you can use them to check your own progress.

Get a Physical

We cannot stress too strongly the importance of a full physical examination before you begin your exercise program. No matter how healthy you may think you are, a physical may uncover latent problems that could give you difficulty in exercising. If your examination does bring a problem to light, your doctor will be able to advise you how to proceed. It's very unlikely that you'll have a medical condition that would preclude exercise, but your doctor may wish to suggest modifications to your exercise program so that you build up your fitness without damage to yourself. A proper physical examination is simply good insurance and a relatively small investment to make for your own physical safety.

Although your regular physician is the best person to determine the form of a medical examination, we would expect it to include a detailed medical history that goes as far back as childhood ailments and injuries. Since you will be putting stress on your heart and lungs, the physical should include electrocardiograms (EKG) at rest, standing, and during and after light exercise. For the older person, a full stress test (see next section) may be advisable. A chest X ray and the usual blood and urine tests should be included in your physical.

Be sure, too, that you explain to your doctor how you intend to exercise. Describe the programs suggested in this book and obtain your physician's approval before you start. As we've often mentioned, interval training programs are easily modified to suit the individual. If your doctor thinks you should go more slowly than we've suggested, it's a simple matter to redesign your own interval training program.

The Exercise Tolerance (Stress) Test

You have no doubt seen photos of middle-aged businessmen striding out on small treadmills while attached to all sorts of medical recording apparatus. Such people are undergoing an exercise tolerance test, more popularly known as a stress test, to measure the heart's ability to pump oxygen to the muscles as they work. The exercise tolerance test is an excellent way of identifying people who stand a high risk of developing heart disease, which could result in heart attack or even death. That's why we suggest a stress test for the over-thirty-five person who has previously led a sedentary life.

30. For men especially, a stress test on a treadmill will help your physician check your heart and lungs before you begin your interval training.

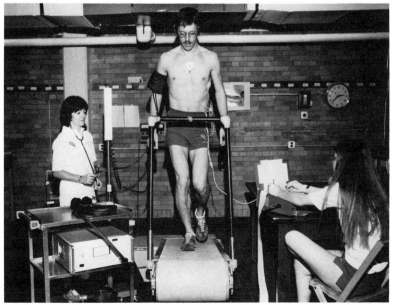

A stress test should be done only after your physician has conducted a conventional physical. Although you can refer yourself to a hospital or clinic with stress-testing facilities, it's best to have your own doctor make the referral. That way, your care can be continued by your own doctor, if necessary. The interpretation of stress test results is also best left to qualified doctors. A negative result does not necessarily mean that you can exercise freely without regard to the load placed on your cardiovascular system. Nor does a positive finding mean that you will need heart surgery or be a cardiac cripple for the rest of your life.

In a typical stress test, the person to be tested is asked to walk on a treadmill while connected to a computerized EKG machine (see photo). The machine records the person's heart rate, blood pressure and the various electrical signals that indicate the working of the heart. One particular part of the EKG tracing shows possible oxygen shortage in the heart muscle, an important factor for anyone who intends to exercise vigorously.

At regular intervals, usually every two or three minutes, the speed and inclination of the treadmill are increased until the person's heart reaches a rate that is determined to be a maximum for his or her age group. However, if certain symptoms develop before the maximal heart rate is reached, the test is stopped and the person allowed to recover. The stress test is arduous and should be done only in a clinic that has not only the proper equipment and staff but also the means to assist patients to recover.

Discuss the results of the stress test with your own doctor. Many people have slight abnormalities of the heart which are disclosed by such tests. However, most abnormalities do not inhibit exercise capability. Nonetheless, take your doctor's advice and follow his or her recommendations as you begin your interval training program.

How to Take Your Own Pulse

An essential part of interval training is making your heart work hard enough during exercise, and the simplest way of checking this is to take your own pulse immediately after a work interval. You should also take your pulse periodically during the rest intervals to check your recovery rate.

Most people are familiar with their pulse in the wrist (see photo), the one traditionally checked by a doctor or nurse during a medical examination. However, if you wish to take your own pulse, you can do so either by placing your hand directly over your left breast or by using two fingers placed gently in front of your ear (see photos). Either of these positions may be easier to use than your wrist. Don't take your pulse using the carotid artery (in the neck), since the pressure from your fingers could cause considerable slowing of the heart rate and might cause cardiac abnormalities.

Using a stopwatch, count the number of beats in six seconds and multiply by 10 to convert to beats per minute. At rest, seven beats in a six-second interval would indicate a heart rate of seventy beats per minute. After exercise, seventeen beats in a six-second interval would show a heart rate of 170

31. The three easiest positions to check your pulse are in the wrist (*left*) directly over the left breast (*center*) or just in front of the ear (*right*). Try each one to see which is the best for you.

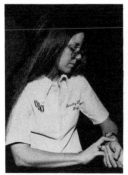
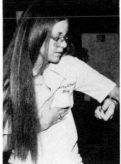
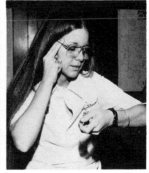

beats per minute. The heart rates you should aim for immediately after exercise are shown in Table 7.

There are alternative ways of taking your pulse, of course. With the rise in the popularity of jogging, a number of electronic devices have appeared that can take your pulse almost instantaneously. The devices are light enough to be carried as you run or bike. However, like many electronic gadgets, the pulse indicators are expensive. We think the manual method is just as effective for interval training.

Watch Your Weight

You should also check your weight as you work through an exercise program. This is especially important if you are restricting your diet in order to lose weight at the same time that you exercise. Once a week is enough, provided you do weigh yourself at the same time and under the same conditions each week. We suggest you check your weight every Monday morning before breakfast. Not only will the weight check be a reminder to control your weekend eating, but it will, we hope, also inspire you to continue with your weight control during the rest of the week.

An ordinary bathroom scale will do for checking your weight. Bathroom scales aren't as accurate as those in a doctor's office, but the readings they give will be sufficiently consistent from week to week. You'll be able to tell if you are losing the couple of pounds or so that we recommend you lose, or are putting on weight.

Two pounds a week is a safe loss of weight for most people. If your scales show that you are losing more than a couple of pounds per week, check with your physician to see if there is some other cause of weight loss (in addition to your dieting). If you are gaining weight, the remedy will usually be up to you: reduce your intake of food, as suggested in Chapter Nine.

Tests for Your Oxygen System

Your oxygen or aerobic system can be measured quite easily with no more than a stopwatch and a bench, though the exercise physiologist now uses very sophisticated equipment (see photo) to measure aerobic energy production.

A simple test you can perform in your own home is to step on and off a bench for as long as possible, at a fixed rate, and then check your pulse during recovery. For men, this test is usually called the Harvard Step Test, since it was developed in the Harvard Fatigue Laboratories during World War II. The women's version of the test is called the Sloan Test, after A. W. Sloan, who modified the Harvard Step Test.

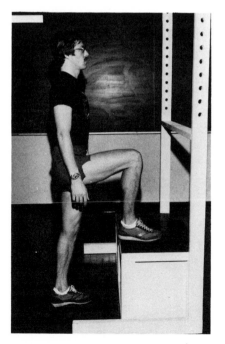

32. The Harvard Step Test is a simple way of checking your oxygen system by stepping on a bench for several minutes and taking your pulse during subsequent recovery.

For the bench test you'll need a bench or a firm chair 20 inches high (17 inches for women). Step up on the bench, one foot at a time, and then down at a rate of thirty steps per minute for as long as you can or for up to five minutes. Take your pulse after stopping, at one-minute intervals (time your pulse for thirty seconds at one, two, and three minutes after exercising). Add the three pulse rates together. You can then compute a fitness index according to this formula:

$$\text{Fitness Index} = \frac{(\text{Time of exercise in seconds}) \times 100}{2 \times (\text{Sum of pulse counts during recovery})}$$

Some standards for various age groups are given in Tables 38 and 39 for men and women. You may be interested to compare yourself to these standards, but we think it's more important to make comparisons of your own fitness. We suggest you try this test before starting an interval training program and then at monthly intervals thereafter. That way, you'll be able to see the changes in your own aerobic conditioning and develop your own standards for yourself.

There are two other useful tests of aerobic conditioning, developed by Dr. Kenneth Cooper, the author of *Aerobics.*

The Harvard Step Test (Men)*

Fitness Index	Under 30	30–50	Over 50
Under 54	Poor	Poor	Poor
54–67	Fair	Average	Good
68–82	Average	Good	Excellent
83–96	Good	Excellent	
Over 96	Excellent		

Table 38   *Based on data from E. L. Fox, C. E. Billings, R. L. Bartels, R. Bason, and D. Mathews: "Fitness Standards for Male College Students," *Int. Z. angew. Physiol. 31*:231–236, 1973.

The Sloan Test (Women)*

Fitness Index	*Under 30*	*30–50*	*Over 50*
Under 55	Poor	Poor	Poor
55–67	Fair	Average	Good
68–79	Average	Good	Excellent
80–90	Good	Excellent	
Over 90	Excellent		

Table 39   *Based on data from A. W. Sloan, "A Modified Harvard Step Test for Women," *J. Appl. Physiol. 14*:985–986, 1959.

Cooper suggests that the distance you can travel by running, swimming, or cycling in twelve minutes correlates very well with your aerobic capacity. Tables 40 and 41 give the guidelines for Cooper's twelve-minute test for running for both men and women. You can calculate the swimming distances by dividing by 4 and the cycling distances by multiplying by 2.5.

Cooper also recommends a test of measuring the time required to cover one and a half miles by running. Table 42 gives the standards for this test for men. (Cooper notes that no separate chart is provided for women because available data are too tentative.) It's up to you which test you use, but we feel that the bench tests are probably the best indicators of aerobic conditioning.

Tests for Your Lactic Acid System

The best way of checking the performance of your lactic acid system is by taking a blood sample immediately following exercise. Measuring the amount of lactic acid in the blood following an all-out exercise lasting between one and a half and two minutes will give an accurate indication of the performance of your lactic acid system. Taking a blood sample

Cooper's 12-minute Test for Running, Swimming and Cycling (Men)*

	Running	
	Under 30	*30–39*
Very poor	Under 1.22 mi.	Under 1.18 mi.
Poor	1.22–1.31	1.18–1.30
Fair	1.32–1.49	1.31–1.45
Good	1.50–1.64	1.46–1.56
Excellent	Over 1.65	Over 1.57

	Swimming	
	Under 30	*30–39*
Very poor	Under 400 yds.	Under 350 yds.
Poor	400–499	350–449
Fair	500–599	450–549
Good	600–699	550–649
Excellent	Over 700	Over 650

	Cycling	
	Under 30	*30–39*
Very poor	Under 2.50 mi.	Under 2.25 mi.
Poor	2.50–3.49	2.25–3.24
Fair	3.50–4.49	3.25–4.24
Good	4.50–5.49	4.25–5.24
Excellent	Over 5.50	Over 5.25

Table 40
*Distances are based on data from K. Cooper: *The Aerobics Way* (New York: M. Evans, 1977), pp. 88, 91, 92.

	40–49	50 and up
	Under 1.14 mi.	Under 1.03 mi.
	1.14–1.24	1.03–1.16
	1.25–1.39	1.17–1.30
	1.40–1.53	1.31–1.44
	Over 1.54	Over 1.45

	40–49	50 and up
	Under 300 yds.	Under 250 yds.
	300–399	250–349
	400–499	350–449
	500–599	450–549
	Over 600	Over 550

	40–49	50 and up
	Under 2.00 mi.	Under 1.75 mi.
	2.00–2.99	1.75–2.49
	3.00–3.99	2.50–3.49
	4.00–4.99	3.50–4.49
	Over 5.00	Over 4.50

Cooper's 12-minute Test for Running, Swimming and Cycling (Women)*

	Running	
	Under 30	*30–39*
Very poor	Under .96 mi.	Under .94 mi.
Poor	.96–1.11	.95–1.05
Fair	1.12–1.22	1.06–1.18
Good	1.23–1.34	1.19–1.29
Excellent	1.35–1.45	1.30–1.39

	Swimming	
	Under 30	*30–39*
Very poor	Under 300 yds.	Under 250 yds.
Poor	300–399	250–349
Fair	400–499	350–449
Good	500–599	450–549
Excellent	Over 600	Over 550

	Cycling	
	Under 30	*30–39*
Very poor	Under 1.5 mi.	Under 1.25 mi.
Poor	1.5–2.49	1.25–2.24
Fair	2.5–3.49	2.25–3.24
Good	3.5–4.49	3.25–4.24
Excellent	Over 4.5	Over 4.25

Table 41
*Distances are based on data from K. Cooper: *The Aerobics Way* (New York: M. Evans, 1977), p. 88, 91, 92.

40–49	50 and up
Under .88 mi.	Under .84 mi.
.88–.98	.84–.93
.99–1.11	.94–1.05
1.12–1.24	1.06–1.18
1.25–1.34	1.19–1.30

40–49	50 and up
Under 200 yds.	Under 150 yds.
200–299	150–249
300–399	250–349
400–499	350–449
Over 500	Over 450

40–49	50 and up
Under 1.0 mi.	Under .75 mi.
1.0–1.99	.75–1.49
2.0–2.99	1.50–2.49
3.0–3.99	2.50–3.49
Over 4.0	Over 3.5

Cooper's 1.5 Mile Test*

	Men	
	Under 30	*30–39*
Very poor	Over 16:01†	Over 16:31†
Poor	14:01–16:00	14:44–16:30
Fair	12:01–14:00	12:31–14:45
Good	10:46–12:00	11:01–12:30
Excellent	Under 10:45	Under 11:00

†Minutes:secs.

	Women	
	Under 30	*30–39*
Very poor	Over 19:01†	Over 19:31†
Poor	18:31–19:00	19:01–19:30
Fair	15:55–18:30	16:31–19:00
Good	13:31–15:54	14:31–16:30
Excellent	12:30–13:30	13:00–14:30

Table 42
  *From K. Cooper, *The Aerobics Way* (New York: M. Evans, 1977), p. 89.
  †Minutes:secs.

50-yard Dash with 15-yard Running Start

	15–20	*20–30*
Poor	Over 7.1*	Over 7.8*
Fair	7.1–6.8	7.8–7.5
Good	6.7–6.5	7.4–7.1
Excellent	Under 6.5	Under 7.1

	15–20	*20–30*
Poor	Over 9.1*	Over 10.0*
Fair	9.1–8.4	10.0–9.2
Good	8.3–7.9	9.1–8.7
Excellent	Under 7.9	Under 8.7

Table 43
  *Seconds.

	40–49	50 and up
	Over 17:31†	Over 19:01†
	15:36–17:30	17:01–19:00
	13:01–15:35	14:31–17:00
	11:31–13:00	12:31–14:30
	Under 11:30	Under 12:30

	40–49	50 and up
	Over 20:01†	Over 20:31†
	19:31–20:00	20:01–20:30
	17:31–19:30	19:01–20:00
	15:56–17:30	16:31–19:00
	13:45–15:55	14:30–16:30

Men		
30–40	40–50	Over 50
Over 9.0*	Over 10.8*	Over 13.0*
9.0–8.6	10.8–10.3	13.0–12.4
8.5–8.1	10.2–9.7	12.3–11.6
Under 8.1	Under 9.7	Under 11.6
Women		
30–40	40–50	Over 50
Over 11.5*	Over 13.8*	Over 16.5*
11.5–10.6	13.8–12.7	16.5–15.2
10.5–10.0	12.6–12.0	15.1–14.4
Under 10.0	Under 12.0	Under 14.4

is hardly practical, but we can suggest a few tests that will give some indication of your performance.

The lactic acid system is the prime source of energy for all-out efforts that last between 90 and 120 seconds, so we can use exercise performances within those times as a personal indicator of lactic acid system capacity. For example, the bench step test can indicate the capacity of the lactic acid system in the large muscles of the thighs and legs. Simply count the number of steps onto a 20-inch bench (17-inch for women) that you can do in one and a half minutes. We can't give you any standards for this test, since your performance will vary according to your skill in doing the exercise, among other factors. As we suggested before, you can use this test to establish your own personal standard and measure yourself against that standard. If your lactic acid system capacity is improving, your standard—that is, the number of steps that you can do in one and a half minutes—should go up as your exercise program continues.

Similarly, you can use your performance times in running, swimming and cycling as a measure of your lactic acid system. For running, we suggest using times in either of three distances—220 yards, 440 yards, and 660 yards. For swimmers, the appropriate distances would be 55 yards, 110 yards and 165 yards. For cyclists, we suggest ½ mile, ¾ mile and 1 mile.

Tests for Your Anaerobic System

Accurate tests of anaerobic capacity are quite difficult. The only reliable method is to measure the amount of ATP in a particular muscle by means of a biopsy (removing small pieces of tissue for pathological analysis). Obviously, a muscle biopsy is impractical. However, there are some less sophisticated methods that can give useful indications of an-aerobic capacity.

The simplest test is the time required to run 50 yards with a 15-yard running start. You'll need a friend with a stopwatch and a marked track to perform this test. Standards for the 50-yard dash for both men and women are shown in Table 43. The results correlate quite well with other, more complex tests.

The Lewis Nomogram for Determining Anaerobic Power from Jump-reach Score and Body Weight

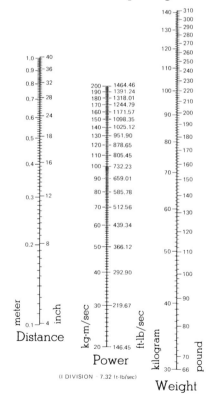

Table 44

A test that is more complicated in execution and interpretation but still possible for the amateur is the jump and reach test. For this test, a blackened plywood board, 5 feet long and 1 foot wide, can be mounted on a basketball backstop or a wall. If mounted on a wall, the board should be at least 6 inches out from the wall so that the jumper does not scrape himself while jumping.

The jumper's hands are first chalked (preferably with magnesium). She then stands on a line one foot out from the board and reaches as high as possible, keeping both heels on the floor. The jumper then does three jumps from a crouched position, making a mark on the board at the top of each jump.

33. You can check your anaerobic capacity with the jump and reach test. The height of your jump and your weight can be used to calculate your power output.

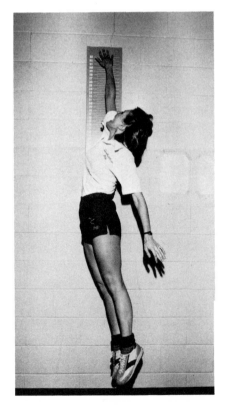

The distance from the top of the reach mark to the top of the highest jump mark is recorded as the score (to the nearest quarter inch).

The jumper's power output can then be calculated from the score and the person's body weight, using a chart known as the Lewis Nomogram (see Table 44). For example, if the jumper weighs 180 pounds and reaches 24 inches, a ruler is laid across the nomogram touching 24 inches on the distance scale (left) and 180 pounds on the weight scale (right). The power output is then read from the center scale—in this case, approximately 1025 foot-pounds/second, or about 1.8 horsepower (to convert ft-lb/sec to HP, multiply by 0.0018).

This is a reliable and relatively easy means of obtaining a person's power output, which is closely related to anaerobic capacity. It is much better than just the distance jumped, because the body weight of the jumper is also considered.

Tests for Strength and Flexibility

Sit-ups and push-ups are not only excellent exercises for building upper-body and stomach muscles; they are also good indicators of muscle strength. Both exercises are described in some detail in Chapter Three.

As a measure of your muscular strength, you can use either bent-knee sit-ups or push-ups or modified push-ups if you can't do the regular variety. Simply count the number of exercises you can do in a two-minute period. If a complete sit-up is done in two seconds (up on count "one," down on count "two"), sixty, which is excellent, can be done in two minutes. Remember that as an exercise to increase the number of continuous sit-ups which may be performed, you can construct your own I.T. prescription, as we suggested in Chapter Seven.

Tables 46 and 47 give guidelines for sit-ups and push-ups according to age group, but remember that these are in-

Sit-ups and Push-ups by Age (Men)

	15–25		26–35		Over 35	
	Sit-ups	Push-ups	Sit-ups	Push-ups	Sit-ups	Push-ups
Minimum	10	8	8	7	5	3
Fair	25	15	20	12	15	8
Good	50	25	40	20	30	15
Excellent	80	40	70	30	50	20

Table 45

Sit-ups and Push-ups by Age (Women)

	15–25		26–35		Over 35	
	Sit-ups	Push-ups*	Sit-ups	Push-ups	Sit-ups	Push-ups
Minimum	5	8	4	7	2	3
Fair	15	15	10	12	5	8
Good	20	25	15	20	10	15
Excellent	30	40	20	30	15	20

Table 46   *Modified push-up.

tended only as a rough guide. The best comparison is between your own pre-training and post-training scores. You should set up your own standards for your own performance.

A simple test of flexibility is to touch the floor without bending the knees. For most people this will be a sufficient test, but it is possible to devise simple equipment for a more precise test of flexibility. One such test is called the Wells Sit and Reach Test. As the name implies, the person being tested sits on the floor and reaches forward, the degree of reach being measured by a yardstick (see photo). The longer the reach, the greater the flexibility.

of myself. I hadn't run sprints like that since leaving high school. Of course, I got a few amazed stares from the guys on the golf course, but nowadays they are so used to my performance that they even say "Good morning" and note my absence if I miss a workout.

I progressed pretty happily through the eight weeks of my own interval training program. I must admit to a few problems, though. The workout that calls for eight 220s (down the field and back, for me) followed by eight 110s is a pretty demanding exercise routine. There have been a few days, principally following evenings that were a mite too convivial, where I may have slipped a second or two in getting through that particular workout. Then there was the day the groundskeeper decided to turn on his full field sprinkler system just as I was in the middle of a run. Wet grass can be like ice and my performance was much like that of a drunken seal on an iceberg. Needless to say, the groundskeeper and I later came to an understanding about such matters.

Now, of course, I'm down to one workout a week, but I enjoy it so much that I usually do two a week, one with longish runs of half and quarter miles and the other with mostly shorter but faster sprints. Even with the rest intervals, my workouts are over in twenty minutes or so, which means I can usually squeeze them in before breakfast. Not only do I feel ready for the day after my workout; I eat a pretty sizable breakfast too.

Has interval training made a difference to me? There's no question but that I'm fitter now than I've ever been. I recently donated some blood at a local hospital and the nurse took my pulse twice because she didn't believe the reading. My resting heart rate is usually below fifty beats a minute, which, I'm told, is very low for a person my age. At my last physical, my doctor said, "I don't have to tell you that there's nothing wrong with you. I think you know it." That doctor is perfectly correct. I know I'm fit because my body tells me so.

There are a few other pleasant side effects. I had to throw out a couple of pairs of pants because my waist has lost a couple of inches. It's not that I've lost any weight, but my stomach muscles are much firmer, so my stomach is where it ought to be and my waist shows it. I even get a few compliments about my shape—and I'm a nonjock, don't forget.

I recently played tennis with an old opponent whom I'd not seen for several months. I'd like to be able to tell you that I beat him, but unfortunately, he's still better at the game than I am. However, when we came off the court my old enemy said, "I've never seen you run so much before. You got to some near-impossible balls so I had to work real hard to beat you." A small victory perhaps, but just another of the satisfying results of my interval training program.

During the summer, I sometimes substitute swimming for part of my running workout. I simply run to the beach, rest, swim with appropriate rests and then jog back home. I guess I could also bicycle, but the running seems to suit me well enough. I don't get bored by the running, since that activity allows me to chew over a few matters in my mind as I run. I'm sure I'd have to concentrate more on traffic and the like if I were on a bicycle.

So you can see that I've become a convert to the idea of interval training. So much so that I decided to collaborate with Drs. Fox and Mathews on this book. Like I said, if interval training can work for me, then it can work for you too. I proved the program to myself, got myself fit and helped write a book at the same time. I expect to continue using interval training for the rest of my life. That's how convinced I am about the method.

I hope that I've convinced you, too, of the merits of interval training. All that's left now is for you to figure out the best program for you and start your training right away. Don't put it off until "everything is just right." Tomorrow morning, set the alarm for a half hour earlier, get out of bed and get started on the first week of your first interval training. The time you spend on getting fit will be the best investment in yourself you have ever made. It's a continuing investment, of course, but the rewards far outweigh the time and effort that it takes to get fit and stay fit.

While you are at it, why not persuade the rest of your family to go along with you? There's no one who's too old or too young to work out using interval training. There's also nothing like a little peer group pressure for making sure that you keep up with the program. Remember the case of the Dorseys, where Helen became fitter than her husband with interval training? A little friendly rivalry in the family might add an extra edge to your training sessions.

And if that isn't enough to keep you on a training program, you might like to think about this: Dr. Richard Stein of Brooklyn's Downstate Medical Center did some intriguing tests on post–heart attack patients who were using interval training to aid their recovery. Dr. Stein's tests suggest that for his patients, interval training helped their performance in the bedroom. There seems to be no reason why we shouldn't conclude that what is good for heart patients isn't also good for all of us. As they say in TV courtroom dramas, "I rest my case."

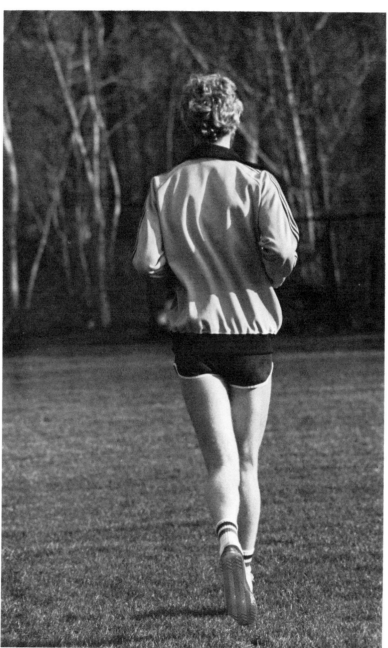

36. (Photo credit: Stephen Szurlej)

INDEX